Keto Diet Cookbook

100 Keto Recipes With Effective 5-Week Meal Plan Diary and Detailed Shopping Lists

Miriam Alley

SPECIAL DISCLAIMER

All the information's included in this book are given for instructive, informational and entertainment purposes, the author can claim to share very good quality recipes but is not headed for the perfect data and uses of the mentioned recipes, in fact the information's are not intent to provide dietary advice without a medical consultancy. The author does not hold any responsibility for errors, omissions or contrary interpretation of the content in this book.

It is recommended to consult a medical practitioner before to approach any kind of diet, especially if you have a particular health situation, the author isn't headed for the responsibility of these situations and everything is under the responsibility of the reader, the author strongly recommend to preserve the health taking all precautions to ensure ingredients are fully cooked.

All the trademarks and brands used in this book are only mentioned to clarify the sources of the information's and to describe better a topic and all the trademarks and brands mentioned own their copyrights and they are not related in any way to this document and to the author.

This document is written to clarify all the information's of publishing purposes and cover any possible issue.

This document is under copyright and it is not possible to reproduce any part of this content in every kind of digital or printable document. All rights reserved.

Table of Contents

Introduction

The keto diet is a low carb diet, abundant source of fats, and shares several similarities with Atkins diets and low sugar diets. This diet involves drastically reducing sugar intake and replacing it with carbohydrates, which is an exceedingly metabolic state known as acetonemia.

When this happens, your body becomes improbably economical at turning fat into energy. It additionally converts fats into ketones within the liver, which may give energy to the brain.

The keto diet has been gaining quality for many years because of its several advantages, as well as weight loss and improved health. In contrast to different fashionable diets, the "keto" isn't a cult and is here to remain. Indeed, several studies have shown the advantages of the keto diet within the context of polygenic disorder, metabolic syndrome, epilepsy, and Alzheimer's illness, among others.

Many keto clinics and diet specialists across the world are currently providing the services of the Keyto consultation. Their goal is to assist folks in winning and maintaining a healthy weight, and in enhancing their polygenic disorder and different metabolic issues through a whole-food approach, no supplements or pre-packaged meals. Dr. Elyssa Elman and Lauren Richer, registered dietitians, are serving to patients for several years to thin and regain their health. They answer a number of the foremost commonly asked questions about the keto diet.

This book has brought a kind of discipline and training for keto diet lovers. Practice around 100 keto diet recipes for 5 weeks, and build a discipline to obtain a healthy diet.

5 Week Meal Plan & Shopping List

Week 1

Days	Breakfast	Lunch	Dinner
Tuesday	Keto Sausage and Biscuits Nutritional values: calories:357 Fats:23.6g Carbs:3.9g Proteins:18g	Keto Caesar salad Nutritional values: calories:1018 Fats:87g Carbs:4g Proteins:51g	Low Carb Taco Casserole Nutritional values: calories:581 Fats:40g Proteins:44g
Wednesday	Keto Breakfast Hot Pockets Nutritional values: calories:640 Fats:50.5g Carbs:7.5g Proteins:39.9g	P.F. Chang's Chicken Lettuce Wraps Nutritional values: calories:366 Fats:20g Carbs:19g Proteins:29g	Asparagus Stuffed Chicken Parmesan Nutritional values: calories:572 Fats:31g Carbs:10g Proteins:62g
Thursday	Ham, Egg and Cheese Muffins Nutritional values: calories:588 Fats:38g Carbs:9g Proteins:48g	Keto Low Carb Chili Recipe - Crock Pot Nutritional values: calories:306 Fats:18g Carbs:13g Proteins:23g	Caprese Hasselback Chicken Nutritional values: calories:365 Fats:21g Carbs:4g Proteins:32g

Friday	Keto Breakfast Sandwich	Keto Tex-Mex casserole	Ham & Smoked Mozzarella Hasselback Chicken
	Nutritional values: calories:603 Fats:54g Carbs:4g Proteins:22g	Nutritional values: calories:751 Fats:57g Carbs:8g Proteins:49g	Nutritional values: calories:336 Fats:18g Carbs:9g Proteins:34g
Saturday	Keto mushroom omelet	Keto Grilled chicken	Caprese Hasselback Chicken
	Nutritional values: calories:517 Fats:5g Carbs:44g Proteins:26g	Nutritional values: calories:690 Fats:25g Carbs:70g Proteins:45g	Nutritional values: calories:365 Fats:21g Carbs:4g Proteins:39g
Sunday	Keto western omelet	Atkins Frozen Crustless Chicken Pot Pie	Keto Chinese pork with Brussels sprouts
	Nutritional values: calories:687 Fats:56g Carbs:6g Proteins:40g	Nutritional values: calories:300 Fats:21g Carbs:9g Proteins:20g	Nutritional values: calories:993 Fats:97g Carbs:7g Proteins:19g

Shopping list

- Green almonds
- Vegetables
- Carrots
- Peppers
- Chicken
- Mushrooms
- Beef
- Spinach
- Avocadoes
- Sausages
- Lettuce leaves
- Cucumbers
- Black olives
- Coconut milk
- Almond milk
- Catfish

Week 2

Days	Breakfast	Lunch	Dinner
Monday	1 cup bullet-proof coffee + 1 cream cheese pancake organic maple syrup	Low Carb Turkey And Pepper	Keto Chicken Zoodles Tomatoes & Spiced Cashews
	Nutritional values: calories:44 0 Fats:50g Carbs:0g Proteins:1g	Nutritional values: calories:230 Fats:8g Carbs:11g Proteins:30g	Nutritional values: calories:411 Fats:18.8g Carbs:11.7g Proteins:45g
Tuesday	Keto frittata with fresh spinach	Asian style stir-fried chicken and veggies	Creamy Tuscan Garlic Chicken
	Nutritional values: calories:66 1 Fats:59g Carbs:4g Proteins:27g	Nutritional values: calories:69 0 Fats:70g Carbs:20g Proteins:45g	Nutritional values: calories:368 Fats:25g Carbs:7g Proteins:30g
Wednesday	Sullivan's keDough breakfast pizza	Keto Chicken Tikka Masala Meatballs	Keto Butter Chicken
	Nutritional values: calories:103 1 Fats:87g Carbs:8g Proteins:53g	Nutritional values: calories:49 5 Fats:41g Carbs:10g Proteins:23g	Nutritional values: calories:293 Fats:17g Carbs:9g Proteins:29g

Thursday	Keto scrambled eggs with halloumi cheese	Keto Ramen, Quick and Easy	Taco Stuffed Avocados
	Nutritional values: calories:657 Fats:59g Carbs:4g Proteins:28g	Nutritional values: calories:306 Fats:19g Carbs:8g Proteins:18g	Nutritional values: calories:410 Fats:g Carbs:15g Proteins:26g
Friday	Keto breakfast tapas	Keto Thai fish curry	Beef and Broccoli Bowls with Sunshine Sauce
	Nutritional values: calories:664 Fats:57g Carbs:5g Proteins:30g	Nutritional values: calories:914 Fats:79g Carbs:10g Proteins:42g	Nutritional values: calories:388 Fats:29g Carbs:14g Proteins:30g
Saturday	Low-carb bacon cheeseburger wraps	Salmon Gremolata with Roasted Vegetables	Keto Fried Rice with Pork (Japanese Chahan)
	Nutritional values: calories:684 Fats:51g Carbs:5g Proteins:48g	Nutritional value: Calories:494 Fats:31g Carbs:12g Proteins:42g	Nutritional values: calories:399 Fats:4g Carbs:12g Proteins:16g

Sunday	Keto pancakes with berries and whipped cream	Super Simple Tuna Fish Salad	Keto Italian cabbage stir-fry
	Nutritional values: calories:424 Fats:39g Carbs:4g Proteins:13g	Nutritional values: calories:563 Fats:30.9g Carbs:37.5g Proteins:41.8g	Nutritional values: calories:968 Fats:88g Carbs:9g Proteins:32g

Shopping list

- Fish
- Lettuce
- Spinach
- Eggs
- Pork
- Salmon
- Avocadoes
- Cabbage
- Vegetables
- Mushrooms
- Chicken breasts

Week 3

Days	Breakfast	Lunch	Dinner
Monday	Keto coconut porridge	Harissa Portobello Mushroom "Tacos"	Oven-baked paprika chicken with rutabaga
	Nutritional values: calories:487 Fats:49g Carbs:4g Proteins:9g	Nutritional values: calories:405 Fats:34.4g Carbs:24g Proteins:10g	Nutritional values: calories:1099 Fats:94g Carbs:16g Proteins:61g
Tuesday	Fabulous low-carb n'oat meal	Keto "Swedish" meatballs in gravy	Low-carb Asian style chicken wings
	Nutritional values: calories:615 Fats:61g Carbs:8g Proteins:10g	Nutritional values: calories:612 Fats:51g Carbs:7g Proteins:31g	Nutritional values: calories:685 Fats:51g Carbs:8g Proteins:46g
Wednesday	Keto Croque Monsieur	Low-carb Hungarian Goulash soup	Keto Buffalo drumsticks with chili aioli
	Nutritional values: calories:1083 Fats:92g Carbs:8g Proteins:54g	Nutritional values: calories:498 Fats:41g Carbs:13g Proteins:17g	Nutritional values: calories:569 Fats:42g Carbs:2g Proteins:42g

Friday	Keto avocado pie	Mussel chowder	Keto harvest pumpkin and sausage soup
	Nutritional values: calories:1130 Fats:107g Carbs:9g Proteins:26g	Nutritional values: calories:698 Fats:64g Carbs:12g Proteins:18g	Nutritional values: calories:777 Fats:70g Carbs:7g Proteins:27g
Saturday	Keto Mexican scrambled eggs	Halloumi burger with rutabaga fries	Butter- aked fish Brussels sprouts and mushrooms
	Nutritional values: calories:229 Fats:18g Carbs:2g Proteins:14g	Nutritional values: calories:1289 Fats:112g Carbs:19g Proteins:46g	Nutritional values: calories: 627 Fats:g Carbs:g Proteins:g
Sunday	Scrambled eggs with basil and butter	Low-carb Philly cheesesteak sandwich	Fish with vegetables baked in foil
	Nutritional values: calories:651 Fats:59g Carbs:3g Proteins:26g	Nutritional values: calories:713 Fats:57g Carbs:9g Proteins:40g	Nutritional values: calories:1146 Fats:95g Carbs:14g Proteins:47g

Shopping list

- Almonds
- Almond milk
- Cheese
- Meatballs
- Chicken
- Honey
- Spinach
- Ghee
- Mushrooms

Week 4

Days	Breakfast	Lunch	Dinner
Monday	Classic Bacon And Eggs Nutritional values: calories:272 Fats:22g Carbs:1g Proteins:15g	Keto pulled pork sandwich Nutritional values: calories:1024 Fats:92g Carbs:10g Proteins:36g	Keto zucchini salmon fritters Nutritional values: calories:523 Fats:45g Carbs:3g Proteins:25g
Tuesday	Low-carb cauliflower cheese Nutritional values: calories:511 Fats:44 Carbs:11 Proteins:17	Slow-cooked keto pork roast with creamy gravy Nutritional values: calories:589 Fats:51g Carbs:3g Proteins:28g	Keto fried chicken broccoli and butter Nutritional values: calories:671 Fats:57g Carbs:6g Proteins:32g
Wednesday	Halloumi burger with rutabaga fries Nutritional values: calories:197 Fats:112g Carbs:19g Proteins:46g	Keto tuna cheese melt Nutritional values: calories:787 Fats:67g Carbs:5g Proteins:38g	Keto chicken nuggets green bean fries and BBQ-mayo Nutritional values: calories:869 Fats:74g Carbs:6g Proteins:41g

Thursday	No-bread keto breakfast sandwich	Low-carb cauliflower pizza with green peppers and olives	Indian keto chicken korma
	Nutritional values: calories:354 Fats:30g Carbs:2g Proteins:20g	Nutritional values: calories:1017 Fats:74g Carbs:16g Proteins:68g	Nutritional values: calories:446 Fats:31g Carbs:4g Proteins:34g
Friday	Keto smoked salmon sandwich	Low-carb Indian lamb stew	Keto salmon with pesto and spinach
	Nutritional values: calories:566 Fats:50g Carbs:3g Proteins:23g	Nutritional values: calories:610 Fats:44g Carbs:16g Proteins:33g	Nutritional values: calories:893 Fats:77g Carbs:3g Proteins:45g
Saturday	Low-carb rutabaga fritters with avocado	Keto sandwich with smoked salmon and horseradish cream	Keto coconut salmon with Napa cabbage
	Nutritional values: calories:950 Fats:87 Carbs:12 Proteins:23	Nutritional values: calories:799 Fats:73g Carbs:4g Proteins:28g	Nutritional values: calories:764 Fats:32g Carbs:3g Proteins:68g
Sunday	Keto Cheese burger	Saffron-flavored fish soup with aioli	Keto salmon pie
	Nutritional values: calories:130 Fats:32g Carbs:10g Proteins:33g	Nutritional values: calories:738 Fats:58g Carbs:12g Proteins:39g	Nutritional values: calories:1056 Fats:97g Carbs:6g Proteins:34g

Shopping list

- Vegetables
- Meatballs
- Rice
- Turkey
- Sardines
- Cauliflower
- Salmon
- Eggs
- Avocadoes
- Tofu

Week 5

Days	Breakfast	Lunch	Dinner
Monday	Keto Egg butter	Keto lamb stew with dill sauce and green beans	Low-carb Sloppy Joes
	Nutritional values: calories:636 Fats:66g Carbs:1g Proteins:12g	Nutritional values: calories:590 Fats:49g Carbs:6g Proteins:29g	Nutritional values: 1073calories: Fats:83g Carbs:15g Proteins:57g
Tuesday	Keto salmon- filled avocados	Keto tortilla with ground beef and salsa	Low-carb eggplant pizza
	Nutritional values: calories:717 Fats:65g Carbs:6g Proteins:22g	Nutritional values: calories:822 Fats:67g Carbs:8g Proteins:42g	Nutritional values: calories:671 Fats:50g Carbs:13g Proteins:37g
Wednesday	Cured salmon with scrambled eggs and chives	Hamburger patties onions and Brussels sprouts	Low-carb Vietnamese pho
	Nutritional values: calories:732 Fats:60g Carbs:2g Proteins:48g	Nutritional values: calories:823 Fats:67g Carbs:12g Proteins:39g	Nutritional values: calories:459 Fats:25g Carbs:13g Proteins:40g

Thursday	Maria's keto Pancakes	Keto meat pie	Keto rutabaga fritters with smoked salmon
	Nutritional values: calories:510 Fats:43g Carbs:2g Proteins:24g	Nutritional values: calories:610 Fats:47g Carbs:7g Proteins:37g	Nutritional values: calories:976 Fats:86g Carbs:11g Proteins:35g
Saturday	Keto egg butter with smoked salmon and avocado	Keto turkey burgers with tomato butter	Keto chops with green beans and avocado
	Nutritional values: calories:1148 Fats:112g Carbs:7g Proteins:13g	Nutritional values: calories:834 Fats:75g Carbs:8g Proteins:33g	Nutritional values: calories:883 Fats:76g Carbs:6g Proteins:38g
Sunday	Keto tuna salad with capers	Keto chicken curry pie	Keto no-noodle chicken soup
	Nutritional values: calories:271 Fats:26g Carbs:1g Proteins:18g	Nutritional values: calories:1142 Fats:105g Carbs:7g Proteins:37g	Nutritional values: calories:509 Fats:40g Carbs:4g Proteins:33g

Shopping list

- avocadoes
- chicken
- broccoli
- banana
- blueberries
- eggs
- turkey chili
- salmon
- lemon
- vegetables

100 Keto Diet Recipes

Breakfast Recipes

1. Keto BLT with cloud bread

25 minutes of preparation 20 minutes of cooking time Servings 2

Ingredients

Cloud bread:
3 eggs
4 oz. cream cheese 1 pinch of salt
½ tablespoon of ground psyllium husk powder
½ tsp baking powder
¼ teaspoon of tartar (optional)

Filling:
4 tbsp mayonnaise
5 oz. bacon
2 ounces lettuce
1 tomato, thinly sliced

Instructions

Cloud bread
Preheat the oven to 300 ° F (150 ° C). Separate the eggs, with egg whites in one bowl and yolks in another. Note, egg whites are better in a metal or ceramic bowl than plastic. Beat the egg whites with salt (and cream of tartar, if using) until very stiff, preferably with a hand mixer.

You should be able to turn the bowl over without the egg whites moving. Add cream cheese, psyllium husk, egg yolks, and baking powder and mix well. Gently fold the egg whites into the egg yolk mixture - try to keep the air in the egg whites. Place two dollops of the mixture per serving on a paper-lined baking tray. Spread the circles with a spatula to about ½ inch (1 cm) thick pieces. Bake in the center of the oven for about 25 minutes, until golden brown.

Building the BLT
Fry the bacon in a frying pan over medium heat until crispy. Place the pieces of sliced bread face down. Spread mayonnaise on any bread. Lay the lettuce, tomato, and bacon in layers between the bread halves.

Nutritional value per serving
Net Carbs: 4% (7 g)
Fiber: 3 g
Fat: 85% (75 g)
Protein: 11% (22 g)
kcal: 800

5 minutes preparation10 minutes of cooking time Portions 1

Ingredients
3 eggs
1 oz. butter, for baking 1 oz. grated cheese
¼ yellow onion, chopped 4 large mushrooms, sliced salt and pepper

Instructions
In a mixing bowl, crack the eggs with a pinch of salt and pepper. Beat the eggs with a fork until smooth and frothy. Melt the butter in a frying pan over medium heat. Add the mushrooms and onion to the pan, stir until tender, then pour in the egg mixture around the vegetables. When the omelet starts to boil and becomes firm, but has a small raw egg left on top, sprinkle cheese over the egg. Use a spatula to gently rub around the edges of the omelet, then fold it in half. When it starts to turn golden brown at the bottom, remove the pan from the heat and slide the omelet onto a plate.

Nutritional value per serving:
Net carbs: 4% (5 g)
Fiber: 1 g
Fats: 76% (44 g)
Protein: 20% (26 g)
kcal: 517

3. Keto frittata with fresh spinach

10 minutes of preparation 35 minutes of cooking time Servings 4

Ingredients
5 oz. diced bacon or chorizo 2 tbsp butter

8 oz. fresh spinach 8 eggs

1 cup of heavy whipping cream 5 oz. grated cheese

Salt and pepper

Instructions
Preheat the oven to 350 ° F (175 ° C). Grease a 9x9 baking dish or individual molds. Fry the bacon until crispy in butter over medium heat. Add the spinach and stir until it has reduced. Remove the pan from the heat and set aside. Beat the eggs and cream together and pour them into the baking dish or ramekins. Add the bacon, spinach, and cheese and place it in the center of the oven. Bake for 25-30 minutes or until set in the center and golden brown on top.

Nutritional value per serving:
Net carbs: 3% (4 g)

Fiber: 1 g

Fats: 81% (59 g)

Protein: 16% (27 g)

kcal: 661

4. Keto browned butter asparagus with creamy eggs

10 minutes of preparation 15 minutes of cooking time Portions 4

Ingredients

2 ounces butter

4 eggs

3 oz. Parmesan cheese, grated

½ cup of sour cream Salt

Cayenne pepper

1½ pounds of green asparagus 1 tbsp olive oil

1½ tbsp lemon juice 3 oz. butter

Instructions

Melt the butter over medium heat and add the eggs. Stir into scrambled eggs. Cook through, but don't overcook the eggs. Spoon the hot eggs into a blender. Add the cheese and sour cream and mix until smooth and creamy. Add salt and cayenne pepper to taste. Toast the asparagus in olive oil over medium heat in a large skillet. Add salt and pepper, remove from skillet and set aside. Fry the butter in the frying pan until it is golden brown and has a nutty aroma. Remove from heat, let cool and add lemon juice. Return the asparagus to the skillet and stir together with the butter until hot. Serve the asparagus with the fried butter and the creamy eggs.

Nutritional value per serving:

Net Carbs: 4% (6 g)

Fiber: 4 g

Fats: 82% (47 g)

Protein: 14% (18 g)

kcal: 518

0 minutes of preparation 10 minutes of cooking time Portions 4

Ingredients
8 eggs
8 tbsp mayonnaise
2 avocados (optional)

Instructions
Bring water to a boil in a saucepan. Optional: make small holes in the eggs with an egg pick. This will help prevent eggs from cracking during cooking. Carefully place the eggs in the water. Boil the eggs for 5–6 minutes for soft-boiled eggs, 6–8 minutes for medium, and 8–10 minutes for hard-boiled eggs. Serve with mayonnaise.

Nutritional value per serving:
Net Carbohydrates: 1% (1 g)
Fiber: 0 g
Fat: 84% (29 g)
Protein: 14% (11 g)
kcal: 316

6. Keto Mexican scrambled eggs

5 minutes preparation 10 minutes of cooking time Portions 4

Ingredients
1 oz. butter
1 spring onion, finely chopped
2 pickled jalapeños, finely chopped 1 tomato, finely chopped
6 eggs
3 oz. grated cheese Salt and pepper

Instructions
Melt the butter in a large skillet over medium heat. Add spring onions, jalapeños, and tomatoes and cook for 3-4 minutes. Beat the eggs and pour them into the pan. Scramble for 2 minutes. Add cheese and herbs.

Nutritional value per serving:
Net Carbohydrates: 3% (2 g)
Fiber: 1 g
Fat: 72% (18 g)
Protein: 24% (14 g)
kcal: 229

7. Keto coconut porridge

0 minutes of preparation 10 minutes of cooking time Portions 1

Ingredients
1 egg, beaten
1 tbsp coconut flour
1 pinch of ground psyllium husk powder 1 pinch of salt
1 oz. butter or coconut oil 4 tbsp coconut cream

Instructions
In a small bowl, combine the egg, coconut flour, psyllium husk powder, and salt. Melt the butter and coconut cream over low heat. Beat in the egg mixture slowly and mix until creamy, thick texture. Serve with coconut milk or cream. Cover your porridge with a few fresh or frozen berries and enjoy!

Nutritional value per serving:
Net carbs: 3% (4 g)
Fiber: 5 g
Fat: 89% (49 g)
Protein: 8% (9 g)
kcal: 487

8. Keto avocado eggs with bacon covers

5 minutes preparation 10 minutes of cooking time Portions 4

Ingredients
2 hard-boiled eggs
½ avocado
1 tsp olive oil 2½ oz. bacon Salt and pepper

Instructions
Preheat the oven to 350 ° F (180 ° C). Place the eggs in a saucepan and cover with water. Bring to a boil and simmer for 8-10 minutes. Immediately place the eggs in ice-cold water when they are cooked to make them easier to peel. Cut the eggs in half lengthwise and scoop out the yolks. Put them in a bowl. Add avocado and oil and mash until combined. Salt and pepper to taste. Place the bacon on a baking tray and fry until crispy. It will take about 5-7 minutes. You can also fry them in a skillet. With a spoon, carefully add the mixture back to the cooked egg whites and turn the bacon off! To enjoy!

Nutritional value per serving:
Net Carbohydrates: 2% (1 g)
Fiber: 2 g
Fat: 83% (14 g)
Protein: 15% (6 g)
kcal: 157

9. Keto scrambled eggs with halloumi cheese

10 minutes of preparation 10 minutes of cooking time Portions 2

Ingredients
2 tbsp olive oil
3 oz. halloumi cheese, cut into cubes 2 spring onions, chopped
4 oz. bacon, cut into cubes
4 tbsp fresh parsley, chopped 4 eggs
Salt and pepper
2 ounces pitted olives

Instructions
Heat olive oil in a frying pan over medium heat and fry the halloumi, spring onions, and bacon until nicely browned. Beat parsley, eggs, salt, and pepper in a small bowl. In the skillet, pour the egg mixture over the bacon and cheese. Reduce heat, add olives, and stir for a few minutes.

Nutritional value per serving:
Net Carbohydrates: 2% (4 g)
Fiber: 1 g
Fats: 81% (59 g)
Protein: 17% (28 g)
kcal: 657

5 minutes preparation 20 minutes of cooking time Portions 4

Ingredients

Pancakes 4 eggs
7 oz. cottage cheese
1 tbsp ground psyllium huskpowder 2 ounces butter or coconut oil
Toppings 2 ounces fresh raspberries or fresh blueberries or fresh strawberries
1 cup of heavy whipping cream

Instructions

Add eggs, cottage cheese, and psyllium husk to a medium bowl and mix. Let sit for 5-10 minutes to thicken up a bit. Heat butter or oil in a non-stick frying pan. Fry the pancakes over medium heat for 3-4 minutes on each side. Don't make them too big or they will be difficult to turn. Add cream to a separate bowl and beat until soft peaks form. Serve the pancakes with the whipped cream and berries of your choice.

Nutritional value per serving:
Net Carbohydrates: 4% (4 g)
Fiber: 3 g
Fats: 83% (39 g)
Protein: 12% (13 g)
kcal: 424

11. Keto Western Omelet

5 minutes preparation 25 minutes of cooking time Portions 2

Ingredients
6 eggs
2 tbsp heavy whipping cream or sour cream Salt and pepper
3 oz. grated cheese, divided 2 ounces butter
5 oz. smoked deli ham, cut into cubes
½ yellow onion, finely chopped
½ green pepper, finely chopped

Instructions
Beat the eggs and cream in a mixing bowl until fluffy. Add salt and pepper. Add half of the grated cheese and mix well. Melt the butter in a large skillet over medium heat. Fry the cubes of ham, onion, and bell pepper for a few minutes. Add the egg mixture and cook until the omelet is almost firm. Be extra careful not to burn the edges. After a while, lower the heat. Sprinkle with the rest of the cheese. Fold the omelet in half if desired. Serve immediately ... and enjoy it!

Nutritional value per serving:
Net carbs: 3% (6 g)
Fiber: 1 g
Fat: 73% (56 g)
Protein: 23% (40 g)
kcal: 687

12. Keto deviled eggs

5 minutes preparation 10 minutes of cooking time Portions 4

Ingredients
4 eggs
1 teaspoon of Tabasco
¼ cup of mayonnaise 1 pinch of herb salt
8 boiled and peeled shrimps or strips of smoked salmon Fresh dill

Instructions
Start cooking the eggs by putting them in a saucepan and covering them with water. Place the pan over medium heat and bring to a boil. Cook for 8-10 minutes to make sure the eggs are hard-boiled. Remove the eggs from the pan and place them in an ice bath for a few minutes before peeling them. Split the eggs in half and scoop out the yolks. Place the egg whites on a plate. Puree the yolks with a fork and add Tabasco, seasoning salt, and homemade mayonnaise. Add the mixture to the egg white with two spoons and top with each shrimp or a piece of smoked salmon. Decorate with dill.

Nutritional value per serving:
Net Carbohydrates: 1% (0.5 g)
Fiber: 0 g
Fat: 83% (15 g)
Protein: 16% (7 g)
kcal: 163

5 minutes preparation
10 minutes of cooking time Portions 2

Ingredients

2 tbsp butter

4 eggs

Salt and pepper

1 oz. smoked deli ham

2 ounces cheddar or provolone or Edam cheese, cut into thick slices

A few drops of Tabasco or Worcestershire sauce (optional)

Instructions

Add butter to a large skillet and place over medium heat. Add the eggs and easily fry them on both sides. Salt and pepper to taste.

Use a fried egg as the basis for any "sandwich". Next, put the ham/pastrami/cold cuts on each stack and then add the cheese. Finish each stack with a fried egg. Leave in the pan, over low heat, if you want the cheese to melt. If necessary, sprinkle a few drops of Tabasco or Worcestershire sauce and serve immediately.

Nutritional value (per serving):

Net Carbohydrates: 2% (2 g)

Fiber: 0 g

Fat: 76% (30 g)

Protein: 23% (20 g)

kcal: 354

14. Keto breakfast tapas

5 minutes preparation
0 minutes of cooking time Portions 4

Ingredients
4 oz. cheddar cheese 8 oz. prosciutto
8 oz. chorizo
½ cup of mayonnaise 4 oz. cucumber
2 ounces Red pepper

Instructions
Cut the cold cuts, cheese, and vegetables into strips or cubes.
Arrange on a plate, serve, and enjoy.

Nutritional value per serving:
Net carbs: 3% (5 g)
Fiber: 1 g
Fats: 79% (57 g)
Protein: 18% (30 g)
kcal: 664

15. Low-carb fried eggs

5 minutes preparation
10 minutes of cooking time Portions 1

Ingredients

3 oz. ground beef or minced lamb or pork, use the leftovers or cook it however you like. You can also use this recipe.
2 eggs
2 ounces grated cheese

Instructions

Preheat the oven to 400 ° F (200 ° C). Arrange the cooked ground beef mixture in a small baking dish. Then make two holes with a spoon and break the eggs in them. Sprinkle with grated cheese. Bake in the oven until the eggs are cooked, about 10-15 minutes. Let it cool down for a while. The eggs and mince become very hot!

Nutritional value per serving:

Net Carbohydrates: 1% (2 g)
Fiber: 0 g
Fat: 65% (35 g)
Protein: 33% (41 g)
kcal: 498

16. Keto smoked salmon sandwich

5 minutes preparation
10 minutes of cooking time Portions 2

Ingredients
Spicy pumpkin bread
2 tbsp pumpkin pie spice 1 tbsp baking powder
1 teaspoon of salt
2 tablespoons of ground psyllium husk powder
½ cup of flax seeds
1¼ cup of almond flour 1¼ cups of coconut flour 1/3 cup of chopped walnuts
1/3 cup pumpkin seeds + extra for topping 3 eggs
½ cup of unsweetened applesauce
¼ cup of coconut oil 14 oz. pumpkin puree
1 tbsp coconut oil or butter for greasing the pan Toppings
4 eggs
2 tbsp heavy whipping cream 2 ounces butter for frying Salt and pepper
1 pinch of chili flakes 2 tbsp butter
1 oz. leafy vegetables 3 oz. smoked salmon

Instructions
Spicy pumpkin bread. Preheat the oven to 400 ° F (200 ° C) and grease a 7-8 inch (about 10 x 18 cm) loaf pan with butter or oil.
Mix all dry ingredients in a bowl. In a separate bowl, stir together egg, applesauce, pumpkin puree, and oil and mix to a smooth batter with the dry ingredients. Pour into the baking dish and sprinkle a tablespoon of pumpkin seeds on top. Bake on the bottom rack for an hour and test with a toothpick. When it comes out clean, it's done. Building the sandwich Beat the eggs and cream in a bowl. Add salt and pepper to taste. Melt the butter in a frying pan over medium heat. Pour in the egg mixture and stir until blended and

cooked through. Remove from heat. Add chili and mix. Use what you already have at home: Tabasco, dried chili flakes, or freshly chopped chili. Toast two slices of the spicy low-carb pumpkin bread, or low-carb bread. Apply a thick layer of butter.

Top with a few lettuce leaves and the scrambled eggs, then add the salmon and some chopped chives.

Nutritional value per serving:
Net Carbohydrates: 2% (3 g)
Fiber: 4 g
Fat: 81% (50 g)
Protein: 16% (23 g)
kcal: 566

0 minutes of preparation 5 minutes of cooking time Portions 1

Ingredients

1 oz. butter

2 eggs

Salt and pepper

Instructions

In a small bowl, crack the eggs and beat with a fork with some salt and pepper. Melt the butter in a non-stick frying pan over medium heat. Watch carefully - the butter must not turn brown! Pour the eggs into the pan and stir for 1-2 minutes, until creamy and cooked just the way you like them. Remember that the eggs are still cooking even after you put them on your plate.

Nutritional value per serving:

Net Carbohydrates: 1% (1 g)

Fiber: 0 g

Fat: 85% (31 g)

Protein: 14% (11 g)

kcal: 327

15 minutes of preparation 40 minutes of cooking time Portions 4

Ingredients

Frittata
1 pound of mushrooms 4 oz. butter
6 spring onions
1 tbsp fresh parsley 1 teaspoon of salt
½ tsp ground black pepper 10 eggs
8 oz. grated cheese 1 cup of mayonnaise
4 oz. leafy vegetables

Vinaigrette
4 tbsp olive oil
1 tbsp white wine vinegar
½ tsp salt
¼ tsp ground black pepper

Instructions

Preheat the oven to 350 ° F (175 ° C). First, make the vinaigrette and set it aside. Cut the mushrooms as desired, small or large - whatever your preference. Fry the mushrooms over medium heat until golden brown with most of the butter. Lower the heat. Keep some butter for greasing the oven dish. Chop the spring onions and mix with the fried mushrooms. Add salt and pepper to taste and mix in the parsley.

Combine eggs, mayonnaise, and cheese in a separate bowl. Salt and pepper to taste. Add the mushrooms and spring onions and pour everything into a well-greased baking dish. Bake for 30-40 minutes or until the frittata turns golden and the eggs are cooked.

Let cool for 5 minutes and serve with leafy greens and the vinaigrette.

Nutritional value per serving:
Net Carbohydrates: 2% (6 g)
Fiber: 2 g
Fat: 86% (105 g)
Protein: 12% (33 g)
kcal: 1097

10 minutes of preparation 0 minutes of cooking time Portions 4

Ingredients

4 oz. tuna in olive oil

½ cup of mayonnaise or vegan mayonnaise 2 tbsp crème fraîche or cream cheese

1 tbsp capers

½ leek, finely chopped

½ tsp chili flakes Salt and pepper

Instructions

Drain the tuna. Mix all ingredients, season with salt, pepper, and chili flakes. You're done!

Nutritional value per serving:

Net Carbohydrates: 1% (1 g)

Fiber: 0 g

Fat: 87% (26 g)

Protein: 12% (8 g)

kcal: 271

2 minutes preparation
10 minutes of cooking time Portions 1

Ingredients

2 eggs
2 tbsp butter
¼ cup of heavy whipping cream 1 tbsp fresh chives, chopped
2 ounces salted salmon Salt and pepper

Instructions

Beat the eggs well. Melt the butter in a saucepan and then stir in the eggs. Add the cream and heat gently while stirring. Simmer the mixture over low heat for a few minutes while stirring constantly to make the eggs creamy. Season with chopped chives, salt, and freshly ground pepper. Serve with a few slices of salted salmon.

Nutritional value per serving:

Net Carbohydrates: 1% (2 g)
Fiber: 0 g
Fat: 73% (60 g)
Protein: 26% (48 g)
kcal: 732

5 minutes preparation 20 minutes of cooking time Portions 6

Ingredients
2 spring onions, finely chopped
5 oz. chopped air-dried chorizo or salami or cooked bacon 12 eggs
2 tablespoons red pesto or green pesto (optional) Salt and pepper
6 oz. grated cheese

Instructions
Preheat the oven to 350°F (175°C). Line a muffin tin with insertable non-stick baking cups or grease a silicone muffin tin with butter. Add spring onions and chorizo to the bottom of the tin. Beat the eggs with pesto, salt, and pepper. Add the cheese and stir. Pour the batter over the spring onions and chorizo. Bake for 15-20 minutes, depending on the size of the muffin tin.

Nutritional value (per serving):
Net Carbohydrates: 2% (2 g)
Fiber: 0 g
Fat: 70% (26 g)
Protein: 28% (23 g)
kcal: 336

10 minutes preparation
15 minutes of cooking time Portions 6

Ingredients
12 eggs
Salt and pepper, to taste 4 oz. cooked bacon

Instructions
Preheat the oven to 400° F (200° C). Place cupcake cases in a muffin tin. Eggs stick easily, even on non-stick surfaces, except silicone molds. Break an egg into any shape and add a filling of your choice. Choose one of our fillings below, or think of your own! We're going for classic crumbled bacon. Season. Bake in the oven for about 15 minutes or until the eggs are tender.

Nutritional value (per serving):
Net Carbohydrates: 2% (1 g)
Fiber: 0 g
Fat: 71% (16 g)
Protein: 27% (13 g)
kcal: 205

5 minutes preparation
45 minutes of cooking time Portions 4

Ingredients
½ leeks
2 ounces green olives 12 eggs
1 cup of heavy whipping cream 7 oz. grated cheese
1 tsp onion powder
3 oz. Cherry tomatoes
1 oz. Parmesan cheese, shredded Salt and pepper

Instructions
Preheat the oven to 400 ° F (200 ° C). Rinse, trim, and thinly slice the leeks. Add to a greased baking dish along with pitted olives.

Add eggs, cream, the larger amount of grated cheese, and onion powder to a medium bowl. Whisk to combine and season with salt and pepper. Pour the egg mixture over the olives and leeks. Add tomatoes and parmesan cheese. Bake in the oven for 30-40 minutes or until golden brown on top and set in the center. Cover with a piece of aluminum foil if the frying pan gets too brown on the edges before cooking.

Nutritional value (per serving):
Net carbs: 3% (5 g)
Fiber: 1 g
Fat: 75% (52 g)
Protein: 21% (33 g)
kcal: 625

24. Keto Italian breakfast dish

10 minutes preparation
50 minutes of cooking time Portions 4

Ingredients

7 oz. Cauliflower
2 ounces butter
12 oz. fresh Italian sausage 8 eggs
1 cup of heavy whipping cream 5 oz. cheddar cheese
¼ cup of fresh basil, chopped Salt and pepper

Instructions

Preheat the oven to 375 ° F (175 ° C). Grease a 20 x 20 cm baking dish. Rinse the cauliflower, cut into bite-sized pieces. Melt butter in a large skillet over medium heat. Add the cauliflower and cook until it begins to soften. Set aside in a bowl. Add sausage to the pan and use a spoon or spatula to break into chunks. Fry the sausage. Season with salt and pepper. Move the sausage and cauliflower to the baking dish. In a large bowl, beat eggs, cream, cheddar cheese until combined, and season with salt and pepper. Pour the egg mixture over the sausage and sprinkle the basil on top. Bake for 30-40 minutes, or until golden brown and completely in the center. If the frying pan is likely to burn before it is cooked, cover it with aluminum foil.

Nutritional value (per serving):

Net carbs: 2% (5 g)
Fiber: 1 g
Fats: 82% (79 g)
Protein: 16% (34 g)
kcal: 875

25. Keto breakfast dish with bacon and mushrooms

10 minutes preparation
45 minutes of cooking time Portions 4

Ingredients
6 oz. mushrooms
10 oz. bacon
2 ounces butter
8 eggs
1 cup of heavy whipping cream 5 oz. grated cheddar cheese
1 tsp onion powder Salt and pepper

Instructions
Preheat the oven to 400 ° F (200 ° C). Trim the mushrooms and cut them into quarters. Cut the bacon into cubes. Fry the bacon and mushrooms in butter in a frying pan over medium heat until golden brown. Season with salt and pepper. Put the contents of the pan in a greased oven dish. Add remaining ingredients to a medium bowl and beat to combine. Season with salt and pepper. Pour the egg mixture over the bacon and mushrooms and bake in the oven for 30-40 minutes or until golden brown and set in the center. Cover with a piece of aluminum foil if the top of the frying pan threatens to burn before it is cooked. Nutritional value (per serving):

Net carbs: 3% (6 g)
Fiber: 1 g
Fats: 83% (81 g)
Protein: 14% (31 g)
kcal: 876

26. Low carb ginger smoothie

5 minutes preparation

0 minutes of cooking time Portions 2

Ingredients

1/3 cup of coconut milk or coconut cream 2/3 cup of water

2 tbsp lime juice

1 oz. frozen spinach

2 tsp fresh ginger, grated

Instructions

Mix all ingredients. Start with 1 tablespoon of lime and increase the amount to taste. Sprinkle with some grated ginger and serve. So good!!

Nutritional value (per serving):

Net carbs: 12% (3 g)

Fiber: 1 g

Fat: 81% (8 g)

Protein: 6% (1 g)

kcal: 82

3 minutes preparation
2 minutes of cooking time Portions 2

Ingredients
14 oz. unsweetened coconut milk 5 oz. fresh strawberries, sliced
1 tbsp lime juice
½ teaspoon of vanilla extract

Instructions
Place all ingredients in a blender and blend until smooth. Using canned coconut milk (let the liquid drain) makes a creamier, more satisfying smoothie. Add more lime juice if desired.

Nutritional value (per serving):

Net Carbs: 9% (10 g)
Fiber: 1 g
Fat: 87% (42 g)
Protein: 4% (5 g)
kcal: 418

28. Golden low-carb granola

10 minutes preparation 1 hour of cooking time Portions 20

Ingredients
8 oz. pecans or hazelnuts or almonds
2½ oz. unsweetened finely chopped coconut 1 cup of sunflower seeds
4 tablespoons of pumpkin seeds 4 tbsp sesame seeds
¾ cup of flaxseed 1 tbsp turmeric
1 tbsp ground cinnamon 2 tsp vanilla extract
½ cup of almond flour 1 cup of water
4 tbsp coconut oil

To serve
10 cups of whole Greek yogurt or coconut cream

Instructions
Preheat the oven to 300 ° F (150 ° C). Coarsely chop the nuts in a food processor or with a sharp knife. Mix all ingredients in a bowl. Spread on a baking tray lined with parchment paper. Roast in the oven for 20 minutes. Make sure to set a timer. Nuts and seeds are heat sensitive and should not be burned. Remove from oven and stir the mixture, then return to the oven for about 20 more minutes. Please check again. When the granola feels almost dry, turn off the heat and let the granola cool in the residual heat of the cooling oven.

Serve the granola with full-fat Greek yogurt with a little vanilla powder and some extra whipped cream if desired. The granola is very nutritious and filling. A third to a half cup goes a long way

Nutritional value (per serving):

Net Carbohydrates: 8% (7 g)
Fiber: 5 g
Fat: 73% (29 g)
Protein: 18% (16 g)
kcal: 358

Prepare 5 minutes
Cooking time for 0 minutes Servings 1

Ingredients
1 cup of canned, unsweetened coconut milk or unsweetened almond milk
1 tablespoon of flaxseed, whole 1 tablespoon of chia seeds
1 tbsp sunflower seeds 1 pinch of salt

Instructions
Combine all ingredients in a small saucepan. Bring to a boil. Reduce heat and simmer until desired consistency. This shouldn't take more than a few minutes. Top with butter and coconut milk - or almond milk and cinnamon - or fresh, unsweetened berries. The possibilities are endless!

Nutritional value (per serving):

Net Carbs: 5% (8 g)
Fiber: 8 g
Fats: 88% (61 g)
Protein: 7% (10 g)
kcal: 615

Preparation 5 minutes
Cooking time 0
Servings 4

Ingredients
8 oz. cheddar or provolone or Edam cheese, sliced 2 ounces butter

Instructions
Place the cheese slices on a large cutting board. Cut butter into slices with a cheese slicer or cut very thin pieces with a knife. Cover each slice of cheese with butter and roll-up. Serve as a snack.

Nutritional value (per serving):

Net Carbohydrates: 2% (2 g)
Fiber: 0 g
Fat: 82% (30 g)
Protein: 16% (13 g)
Kcal: 331

31. Butter coffee

5 minutes preparation
0 minutes of cooking time Portions 1

Ingredients

1 cup of hot coffee, freshly brewed 2 tbsp unsalted butter
1 tbsp MCT oil or coconut oil

Instructions

Combine all ingredients in a blender. Blend until smooth and foamy.
Serve immediately.

Nutritional value (per serving):

Net Carbohydrates: 0% (0 g)
Fiber: 0 g
Fat: 99% (38 g)
Protein: 1% (1 g)
Kcal: 334

5 minutes preparation
0 minutes cooking time Portions 1

Ingredients
¾ cup of coffee, brewed the way you like it
¼ cup of heavy whipping cream

Instructions
Brew your coffee the way you like it. Pour the cream into a small saucepan and heat gently while stirring until foamy. Pour the warm cream into a large cup, add coffee and stir. Serve immediately as is, or with a handful of nuts or a piece of cheese.

Nutritional value (per serving):
Net Carbohydrates: 3% (2 g)
Fiber: 0 g
Fat: 93% (21 g)
Protein: 4% (2 g)
Kcal: 202

33. Salad sandwiches

5 minutes preparation
0 minutes of cooking time Portions 1

Ingredients
2 ounces Romaine lettuce or baby gem lettuce
½ oz. butter or mayonnaise
1 oz. Edam cheese or other cheese as desired
½ avocado, sliced
4 cherry tomatoes, sliced

Instructions
Rinse the lettuce well and use it as the base for the toppings. Divide butter or mayonnaise over the salad leaves and top with the cheese, avocado, and tomato. To enjoy!

Nutritional value (per serving):
Net carbs: 5% (5 g)
Fiber: 9 g
Fat: 84% (34 g)
Protein: 11% (10 g)
Kcal: 383

5 minutes preparation
0 minutes of cooking time Portions 1

Ingredients

1 oz. unsalted butter
1 teaspoon pumpkin pie spice 2 tsp instant coffee powder
1 cup of boiling water

Instructions

Place butter, spices, and instant coffee in a deep bowl for use with a hand blender. Alternatively, you can put the ingredients directly into a blender jar. Add boiling water and blend for 20-30 seconds until a fine foam is formed. Pour into a cup and sprinkle with some cinnamon or pumpkin spice. Serve immediately! It's even better with a dollop of whipped cream on top.

Nutritional value (per serving):

Net Carbohydrates: 2% (1 g)
Fiber: 1 g
Fat: 97% (23 g)
Protein: 1% (0.5 g)
Kcal: 216

Lunch

35.Keto meat pie

30 minutes of preparation 40 minutes of cooking time Portions 6

Ingredients
Pie crust
¾ cup of almond flour 4 tbsp sesame seeds

4 tbsp coconut flour

1 tbsp ground psyllium husk powder 1 tsp baking powder

1 pinch of salt

3 tbsp olive or coconut oil, melted 1 egg

4 tbsp water

Topping
8 oz. cottage cheese 7 oz. grated cheese

Stuffing
½ yellow onion, finely chopped 1 clove of garlic, finely chopped 2 tbsp butter or olive oil

1¼ pound ground beef or lamb

1 tbsp dried oregano or dried basil salt and pepper

4 tablespoons of tomato paste or ajvar sauce

½ cup of water

Instructions

Preheat the oven to 350 ° F (175 ° C). Fry the onion and garlic in butter or olive oil over medium heat for a few minutes, until the onion is soft. Add ground beef and continue to fry. Add oregano or basil. Salt and pepper to taste. Add tomato paste or ajvar sauce. Add water. Reduce heat and simmer for at least 20 minutes. While the meat is simmering, prepare the dough for the crust.

Mix all crust ingredients in a food processor for a few minutes until the dough forms a ball. If you don't have a food processor, you can mix it by hand with a fork. Place a round piece of parchment paper in a well-greased springform pan or a deep 9-10 inch (23-25 cm) diameter cake pan to make it easier to remove the cake once cooked. Divide the dough in the pan and along the sides. Use a spatula or well-greased fingers.

Once the crust has formed into the pan, poke the bottom of the crust with a fork. Pre-bake the crust for 10-15 minutes. Remove from the oven and place the meat in the crust. Mix cottage cheese and grated cheese and place it on the cake. Bake on the bottom rack for 30-40 minutes or until the pie turns golden.

Nutritional value per serving:

Net Carbs: 4% (7 g)
Fiber: 6 g
Fats: 71% (47 g)
Protein: 25% (37 g)
kcal: 610

36. Keto avocado pie

25 minutes of preparation

40 minutes of cooking time Portions 6

Ingredients
Pie crust

¾ cup of almond flour

¼ cup of sesame seeds

¼ cup of coconut flour

1 tbsp ground psyllium husk powder 1 tsp baking powder

1 pinch of salt

3 tbsp olive oil or coconut oil 1 egg

¼ cup of water

Stuffing
2 ripe avocados

1 cup of mayonnaise 3 eggs

2 tbsp fresh cilantro, finely chopped 1 red chili pepper, finely chopped

½ tsp onion powder

¼ teaspoon of salt 4 oz. cream cheese 5 oz. grated cheese

Instructions
Preheat the oven to 350 ° F (175 ° C). Mix all the ingredients for the pie dough in a food processor for a few minutes until the dough forms a ball. If you don't have a food processor, simply knead the ingredients together in a bowl with a fork or your hands.

Attach a piece of baking paper to a springform tin with a diameter of no more than 26 cm. The springform makes it easier to remove the cake when it is cooked. Grease the pen and paper. Spread the dough in the pan. Use an oiled spatula or your fingers. Pre-bake the crust for 10-15 minutes. Divide the avocado. Remove the peel and stone and cut it into cubes. Remove the seeds from the chili and chop them finely. Place the avocado and chili in a bowl and mix with the other ingredients.

Pour the mixture into the pie crust. Bake for 35 minutes or until lightly golden brown. Let cool for a few minutes and serve with a green salad.

Nutritional value per serving:
Net Carbs: 3% (9 g)
Fiber: 14 g
Fats: 88% (107 g)
Protein: 9% (26 g)
kcal: 1130

37. Keto salmon pie

15 minutes of preparation 40 minutes of cooking time Portions 4

Ingredients
Pie crust
¾ cup of almond flour 4 tbsp sesame seeds
4 tbsp coconut flour
1 tbsp ground psyllium husk powder 1 tsp baking powder

1 pinch of salt
3 tbsp olive oil or coconut oil 1 egg
4 tbsp water

Stuffing
8 oz. smoked salmon 1 cup of mayonnaise 3 eggs
2 tbsp fresh dill, finely chopped
½ tsp onion powder
¼ tsp ground black pepper 5 oz. cream cheese
5 oz. grated cheese

Instructions
Preheat the oven to 350 ° F (175 ° C). Place the ingredients for the pie dough in a food processor with a plastic dough knife. Pulse until the mixture forms a ball. If you don't have a food processor, you can use a fork to mix the dough.

Place a piece of parchment paper in a 10 inch (23 cm) springform pan. (This makes it a cinch to remove once cooked.) Coat your fingers or a spatula and gently press the dough into the springform. Pre-bake the crust for 10-15 minutes, or until lightly browned. Mix all the ingredients for the filling, except the salmon, and pour it into the pie crust. Add the salmon and bake for 35 minutes or until the pie is golden brown. Let cool for a few minutes and serve with a salad or other vegetables.

Nutritional value per serving:

Net Carbohydrates: 2% (6 g)

Fiber: 7 g

Fats: 84% (97 g)

Protein: 13% (34 g)

kcal: 1056

38. Keto chicken curry pie

25 minutes of preparation 40 minutes of cooking time Portions 4

Ingredients
Pie crust
¾ cup of almond flour 4 tbsp sesame seeds
4 tbsp coconut flour
1 tbsp ground psyllium husk powder 1 tsp baking powder
1 pinch of salt
3 tbsp olive oil or coconut oil 1 egg
4 tbsp water

Stuffing

11 oz. boiled chicken 1 cup of mayonnaise 3 eggs
½ green pepper, finely chopped 1 tbsp curry powder
1 tsp paprika powder 1 tsp onion powder
¼ tsp ground black pepper 4 oz. cream cheese
5 oz. grated cheese

Instructions
Preheat the oven to 350 ° F (175 ° C). Put all the ingredients for the pie crust in a food processor for a few minutes until the dough forms a ball. If you don't have a food processor, you can also mix the dough with a fork or by hand. Attach a piece of parchment paper to a springform pan no larger than 10 inches (23 cm) in diameter (the springform makes it easier to remove the cake when it is ready). Grease the bottom and sides of the pan.

Divide the dough in the pan. Use an oiled spatula or your fingers. Pre-bake the crust for 10-15 minutes. Mix all other ingredients before filling and fill the pie base. Bake for 35-40 minutes or until the pie has turned a nice golden brown. Let it cool before serving

Nutritional value per serving:

Net Carbohydrates: 2% (7 g)

Fiber: 8 g

Fat: 84% (105 g)

Protein: 13% (37 g)

kcal: 1142

25 minutes of preparation 40 minutes of cooking time Portions 4

Ingredients
Pie crust
¾ cup of almond flour
¼ cup of sesame seeds
¼ cup of coconut flour

1 tbsp ground psyllium husk powder 1 tsp baking powder
1 pinch of salt
3 tbsp olive oil or coconut oil 1 egg
¼ cup of water

Stuffing
2 ripe avocados
1 cup of mayonnaise 3 eggs
2 tbsp fresh cilantro, finely chopped 1 red chili pepper, finely chopped
½ tsp onion powder
¼ teaspoon of salt 4 oz. cream cheese 5 oz. grated cheese

Instructions
Preheat the oven to 350 ° F (175 ° C). Mix all the ingredients for the pie dough in a food processor for a few minutes until the dough forms a ball. If you don't have a food processor, simply knead the ingredients together in a bowl with a fork or your hands. Attach a piece of baking paper to a springform tin with a diameter of no more than 26 cm. The springform makes it easier to remove the cake when it is cooked. Grease the Pan and paper.

Spread the dough in the pan. Use an oiled spatula or your fingers. Pre-bake the crust for 10-15 minutes. Divide the avocado. Remove the peel and stone and cut it into cubes. Remove the seeds from the chili and chop them finely. Place the avocado and chili in a bowl and mix with the other ingredients.

Pour the mixture into the pie crust. Bake for 35 minutes or until lightly golden brown. Let cool for a few minutes and serve with a green salad.

Nutritional value per serving:
Net Carbs: 3% (9 g)
Fiber: 14 g
Fats: 88% (107 g)
Protein: 9% (26 g)
kcal: 1130

40. Low-carb salad of baked kale and broccoli

5 minutes preparation 15 minutes of cooking time Portions 2

Ingredients
½ cup of mayonnaise
1 tablespoon of whole-grain mustard 4 eggs
½ pound of broccoli 4 oz. Kale
2 spring onions 2 tbsp olive oil
2 cloves of garlic 2 avocados
1 pinch of chili flakes Salt or pepper to taste

Instructions
Combine mayo and mustard in a small bowl and set aside.
Cook the eggs however you like: soft, medium or hard- boiled.
Immediately place them in ice-cold water when cooked through so
that they are easier to peel. After cooling - divide into halves or
quarters. Slice the avocados, remove the stone, and slice them.

Cut the garlic into thin slices. Heat the oil in a frying pan and gently
fry the slices. Remove the garlic from the pan and place on kitchen
paper to make it crispy. Keep the oil in the pan. Coarsely chop
broccoli and kale. Add a knob of butter to the garlic-infused oil in
the pan and sauté the vegetables over medium heat for a few
minutes until soft.

Season with salt and pepper and plate with avocado, eggs, and the
mustard mayonnaise. Top the dish with baked garlic slices for extra
flavor and crunch.

Nutritional value per serving:
Net Carbs: 5% (13 g)
Fiber: 19 g
Fat: 86% (94 g)
Protein: 9% (22 g)
kcal: 1022

20 minutes of preparation 15 minutes of cooking time Portions 4

Ingredients

Dressing
2 tbsp olive oil
¾ cup of mayonnaise or vegan mayonnaise 2 tsp lemon juice
1 clove of garlic, finely chopped
½ tsp salt
¼ tsp chili powder

Salad
1 head of cos lettuce 4 oz. arugula lettuce
¼ cup of finely chopped fresh chives or spring onions 2 courgettes
1 tbsp olive oil salt and pepper
3½ oz. chopped walnuts or pecans

Instructions

Beat all the ingredients for the dressing in a small bowl. Keep the dressing to develop flavor while you make the salad. Trim the salad and cut it into pieces. Place the Romaine, arugula, and chives in a large bowl. Split the zucchini lengthwise and scoop out the seeds. Cut the zucchini halves crosswise into half-inch pieces. Heat olive oil in a skillet over medium heat until it shimmers. Add zucchini to the pan and season with salt and pepper. Sauté until lightly brown but still firm.

Add the cooked zucchini to the salad and mix well. Briefly toast the nuts in the same pan as the zucchini. Season with salt and pepper. Spoon the nuts on the salad and drizzle with salad dressing.

Nutritional value per serving:

Net Carbohydrates: 6% (8 g)

Fiber: 7 g

Fat: 88% (58 g)

Protein: 6% (9 g)

kcal: 595

10 minutes of preparation 20 minutes of cooking time Portions 4

Ingredients
8 oz. goat cheese 8 oz. bacon

2 avocados

4 oz. arugula lettuce 4 oz. walnuts

Dressing
1 tbsp lemons, the juice

½ cup of mayonnaise

½ cup of olive oil

2 tbsp heavy whipping cream Salt and pepper

Instructions
Preheat the oven to 400 ° F (200 ° C) and place baking paper in an oven dish. Cut the goat cheese into half-inch (~ 1 cm) round slices and place it in the baking dish. Fry them on the top rack until golden brown. Fry the bacon until crispy in a pan. Cut the avocado into pieces and put them on the arugula. Add the fried bacon and goat cheese. Sprinkle with nuts

Use a hand blender to make the dressing with the lemon juice, mayonnaise, olive oil, and cream. Season with salt and pepper

Nutritional value per serving:
Net Carbohydrates: 2% (6 g)

Fiber: 9 g

Fats: 89% (123 g)

Protein: 9% (27 g)

kcal: 1251

10 minutes of preparation 45 minutes of cooking time Portions 6

Ingredients
Pie crust
1¼ cup of almond flour 4 tbsp sesame seeds
1 tbsp ground psyllium husk powder
½ tsp salt 1 egg
2 ounces butter

Stuffing
1 oz. butter
2/3 lb smoked pork belly or bacon or pancetta 1 yellow onion
1 tsp dried thyme
½ tsp salt
¼ tsp ground black pepper
1 cup of heavy whipping cream
8 oz. grated cheese 5 eggs

Instructions
Preheat the oven to 350 ° F (175 ° C). Mix all ingredients with the pie crust in a food processor to a firm dough. Divide the dough into a springform pan with well-oiled hands or a spatula. Place baking paper between the ring and the bottom to the baked   cake easier separately to make. Leave it in the refrigerator while you prepare the filling.

Chop the onion and cut the bacon into cubes. Fry in butter until onion and bacon have a nice color. Add spices and stir. Add to the pie crust. Beat the remaining ingredients together and pour them over. Bake on the middle rack for 45 minutes or until the pie is nicely colored. Test with a knife to make sure the egg mixture is firm if unsure

Nutritional value per serving:
Net carbs: 2% (5 g)
Fiber: 3 g
Fats: 86% (83 g)
Protein: 12% (26 g)
kcal: 886

15 minutes of preparation 20 minutes of cooking time Portions 4

Ingredients

Stuffing

2 tbsp butter

2 cloves of garlic, finely chopped 1 shallot, finely chopped

3 oz. mushrooms

5 oz. bacon

2 ounces fresh spinach

2 ounces Parmesan cheese, grated 5 oz. cream cheese

½ tsp salt

¼ teaspoon of pepper Pierogi dough

½ cup of almond flour

¼ cup of coconut flour

½ tsp salt

1 tsp baking powder 6 oz. grated cheese 3 oz. butter

1 egg

1 beaten egg, to coat the top of the pierogi

Instructions

Start with the filling. Sauté shallot, garlic, bacon, mushrooms, and spinach in butter until nicely colored. Salt and Pepper. Reduce heat and add cream cheese and parmesan cheese. Stir and let simmer for another minute. Set aside and let cool. Preheat the oven to 350 ° F (175 ° C). Mix all dry ingredients in a bowl.

Melt the butter and cheese together in a pan over low heat. Stir well for a smooth batter. Remove from heat. Break the egg into the mixture and keep stirring. Add the dry ingredients and mix into a firm dough.

Divide the dough into four balls and use a rolling pin to flatten them into four round pieces about ⅕ inch (½ cm) thin and 7 inches (18 cm) in diameter. Apply a generous amount of filling to each piece of dough, but only half of each piece.

Fold and seal the edges with a fork or your fingers. Brush with a beaten egg and bake for 20 minutes until the pierogis turn golden brown. Serve with a salad and dressing.

Nutritional value per serving:
Net Carbs: 4% (8 g)
Fiber: 5 g
Fats: 82% (79 g)
Protein: 15% (32 g)
kcal: 873

10 minutes of preparation 20 minutes of cooking time Portions 4

Ingredients
Salmon burgers
1½ pounds of salmon 1 egg
½ yellow onion
1 teaspoon of salt
½ tsp pepper
2 ounces butter, for baking Green puree
1 pound of broccoli
5 oz. butter
2 ounces grated Parmesan cheese Salt and pepper to taste
Lemon butter
4 oz. butter at room temperature 2 tbsp lemon juice
Salt and pepper to taste

Instructions
Preheat the oven to 220 ° F (100 ° C). Cut the fish into small pieces and put them in a food processor along with the rest of the ingredients for the burger. Pulse for 30-45 seconds until you have a coarse mixture. Don't mix too well, this can make the burgers hard. Form 6-8 burgers and fry for 4-5 minutes on each side over medium heat in plenty of butter or oil. Keep warm in the oven.

Cut the broccoli into small florets. You can also use the stem, peel it and chop it into small pieces. Bring a pan of lightly salted water to a boil and add the broccoli. Cook for a few minutes until soft, but only when all texture is gone. Drain and discard the boiling water. Use a hand blender or food processor to mix the broccoli with butter and parmesan cheese. Season with Salt and Pepper.

Make the lemon butter by mixing the butter (at room temperature) with lemon juice, salt, and pepper in a small bowl using electric beaters. Serve the warm burgers with a side of green puree and a melting dollop of fresh lemon butter on top.

Nutritional value per serving:
Net carbs: 3% (7 g)
Fiber: 3 g
Fat: 80% (91 g)
Protein: 18% (45 g)
kcal: 1030

10 minutes of preparation 30 minutes of cooking time Portions 4

Ingredients
Chicken patties
1½ pounds of ground turkey or chicken 1 egg
½ yellow onion, grated or finely chopped 1 teaspoon kosher or ground sea salt
½ tsp ground black pepper
1 tsp dried thyme or ground coriander seeds 2 ounces butter, for baking
Baked cabbage
1½ pounds of green cabbage 3 oz. butter
1 teaspoon of salt
½ tsp ground black pepper Whipped tomato butter
4 oz. butter
1 tbsp tomato paste
1 tsp red wine vinegar (optional) Sea salt and pepper to taste

Instructions
Preheat the oven to 220 ° F (100 ° C). Mix all the ingredients for the patties in a bowl. Using wet hands, shape the ground turkey into patties. Fry in butter over medium heat until golden brown and done. Place in the oven to keep warm. Chop the cabbage with a sharp knife, mandolin slicer, or food processor.

Sauté the cabbage in a generous amount of butter over medium heat until brown around the edges, but still has somebody. Stir occasionally to make sure it cooks evenly. Season with Salt and Pepper. Lower the heat towards the end. Put all the ingredients for the tomato butter in a small bowl and beat them together with an electric hand mixer. Place the turkey patties and baked cabbage on a plate and top with a dollop of tomato butter.

Nutritional value per serving:

Net Carbs: 4% (8 g)

Fiber: 5 g

Fat: 80% (75 g)

Protein: 16% (33 g)

kcal: 834

47. Keto spinach and goat cheese pie

30 minutes of preparation 40 minutes of cooking time Portions 6

Ingredients
Egg batter 5 eggs
1 cup of heavy whipping cream or sour cream Salt and pepper
Spinach and goat cheese filling 7 oz. fresh spinach
2 tbsp butter or coconut oil 1 clove of garlic
1 pinch of nutmeg Salt and pepper
3½ oz. grated cheese
6 oz. goat cheese, sliced Pie crust
1¼ cup of almond flour 3 tbsp sesame seeds
1 tbsp ground psyllium husk powder
½ tsp salt 1½ oz. butter 1 egg

Instructions
Preheat the oven to 350° F (175° C). Mix almond flour and sesame seeds in a blender. Add the remaining ingredients and mix into a dough. Press the dough into a springform pan and pierce with a fork. Pre-bake the pie pan for 10-15 minutes. Beat the eggs and whipped cream or sour cream together. Add salt and pepper.

Coarsely chop the spinach. Finely chop the garlic. Fry the garlic in butter or oil, add the spinach and fry a little more. Then Season. Add the chopped spinach to the pre-baked pie pan. Mix the grated cheese into the egg batter and pour the spinach over   it. Top with goat cheese. Bake at 350 ° F (175 ° C) for 30-40 minutes.

Nutritional value per serving:
Net carbs: 3% (4 g)
Fiber: 3 g
Fat: 82% (57 g)
Protein: 15% (23 g)
kcal: 631

15 minutes of preparation

20 minutes of cooking time Portions 2

Ingredients
¾ pound of chicken breasts, bone, and skin 1 tbsp olive oil

Salt and pepper 3 oz. bacon

7 oz. Roman lettuce

1 oz. Parmesan cheese, freshly grated

Dressing
½ cup of mayonnaise 1 tbsp Dijon mustard

½ lemon, zest, and juice

½ oz. grated Parmesan cheese, finely grated

2 tablespoons of finely chopped anchovy fillets 1 clove of garlic, pressed or finely chopped Salt and pepper

Instructions
Preheat the oven to 350 ° F (175 ° C). Mix the ingredients for the dressing with a whisk or hand blender. Set aside in the refrigerator. Place the chicken breasts in a greased oven dish. Season the chicken with salt and pepper and drizzle with olive oil or melted butter. Bake the chicken in the oven for about 20 minutes or until cooked through. You can also cook the chicken on the stove if you prefer.

Fry the bacon until crispy. Finely chop the lettuce and place on two plates as a base. Top with the sliced chicken and crispy crumbled bacon. Finish with a large dollop of dressing and a generous grater of Parmesan cheese.

Nutritional value per serving:

Net Carbohydrates: 2% (4 g)

Fiber: 3 g

Fat: 78% (87 g)

Protein: 20% (51 g)

kcal: 1018

49. Keto Creamy Cheddar Bacon Chicken

Prep time: 0 hours 20 min.
Total time: 3 hours 0 min.
6 serves

Ingredients
1/2 cup low sodium chicken stock 1 tbsp. dried parsley
2 teaspoons dried dill 1 tsp. dried chives 1/2 tsp. onion powder 1/4 tsp. garlic powder
2 lbs chicken breasts boneless Kosher salt
Freshly ground black pepper
2 (8-oz) Blocks of cream cheese, cubed 2 1/4 c shredded cheddar, divided
8 slices of cooked bacon, crumbled Chopped chives, to serve

Travel directions
Pour chicken stock into a 4-liter slow cooker and stir in dried parsley, dill, chives, onion powder, and garlic powder. Add half of the chicken and season with salt and pepper.

Repeat with the remaining half of the chicken. Stir to coat the chicken and set on low for 6 hours or on high for 2 hours. Use two forks to shred the chicken in the slow cooker. Stir in the cream cheese and 2 cups of cheddar cheese until melted. Cover with the remaining 1/4 cup of cheddar, bacon, and chives before serving

Nutritional value (per serving):
Net Carbs: 3% (9 g)
Fiber: 2 g
Fat: 76% (102 g)
Protein: 21% (62 g)
kcal: 1194

5 minutes preparation

0 minutes of cooking time Portions 2

Ingredients

1 lb rotisserie chicken 7 oz. feta cheese

2 tomatoes

2 ounces lettuce

10 black olives

1/3 cup of olive oil Salt and pepper

Instructions

Slice the tomatoes and place on a plate along with chicken, feta cheese, lettuce, and olives. Season with Salt and Pepper. Serve with olive oil.

Nutritional value (per serving):

Net Carbs: 3% (9 g)

Fiber: 2 g

Fat: 76% (102 g)

Protein: 21% (62 g)

kcal: 1194

5 minutes preparation

0 minutes cooking time Portions 2

Ingredients

6 oz. Deli Turkey 1 avocado, sliced

2 ounces lettuce

3 oz. cream cheese 4 tbsp olive oil Salt and pepper

Instructions

Place the turkey, avocado, lettuce, and cream cheese on a plate. Drizzle olive oil over the vegetables and season with salt and pepper.

Nutritional value (per serving):

Net Carbs: 4% (7 g)

Fiber: 7 g

Fat: 82% (60 g)

Protein: 13% (22 g)

kcal: 660

52. Keto smoked salmon plate

5 minutes preparation 0 minutes cooking time Portions 3

Ingredients

¾ pound of smoked salmon 1 cup of mayonnaise

2 ounces baby spinach 1 tbsp olive oil

½ limes (optional) Salt and pepper

Instructions

Place the salmon, spinach, a wedge of lime, and a large dollop of mayonnaise on a plate. Drizzle olive oil over the vegetables and season to taste with salt and pepper.

Nutritional value (per serving):

Net Carbohydrates: 0% (1 g)

Fiber: 1 g

Fat: 86% (97 g)

Protein: 13% (33 g)

kcal: 1016

2 minutes preparation
10 minutes of cooking time Portions 1

Ingredients

2 eggs
2 tbsp butter
¼ cup of heavy whipping cream 1 tbsp fresh chives, chopped
2 ounces salted salmon Salt and pepper

Instructions

Beat the eggs well. Melt the butter in a saucepan and then stir in the eggs. Add the cream and heat gently while stirring. Simmer the mixture over low heat for a few minutes while stirring constantly to make the eggs creamy. Season with chopped chives, salt, and freshly ground pepper. Serve with a few slices of salted salmon.

Nutritional value (per serving):

Net Carbohydrates: 1% (2 g)
Fiber: 0 g
Fat: 73% (60 g)
Protein: 26% (48 g)
kcal: 732

5 minutes preparation
10 minutes of cooking time
Portions 4

Ingredients
9 oz. Brie cheese or Camembert cheese 1 clove of garlic, chopped
1 tbsp fresh rosemary, roughly chopped
2 ounces pecans or walnuts, roughly chopped
1 tbsp olive oil Salt and pepper

Instructions
Preheat the oven to 400 ° F (200 ° C). Place the cheese on a baking tray lined with parchment paper or in a small non-stick baking dish. In a small bowl, combine the garlic, herbs, and nuts along with the olive oil. Add salt and pepper to taste.

Place the nut mixture on top of the cheese and bake for 10 minutes or until the cheese is warm and soft and the nuts are toasted. Serve warm or lukewarm.

Nutritional value (per serving):
Net Carbohydrates: 1% (1 g)
Fiber: 1 g
Fat: 82% (31 g)
Protein: 17% (15 g)
kcal: 342

5 minutes preparation

10 minutes of cooking time Portions 4

Ingredients

8 lamb chops

1 tbsp butter

1 tbsp olive oil Salt and pepper

To serve

4 oz. herb butter

1 lemon, in wedges

Instructions

Let the pork chops come to room temperature before baking or grilling. The meat should not be cold when cooked; otherwise, it will not have a nice brown surface. If you make a few cuts in the fat area, the heel will not curl up. Season with Salt and Pepper.

Fry in butter and some olive oil if using a skillet. If you're grilling, just brush some olive oil before putting the chops on the grill. Fry them for 3-4 minutes, depending on how thick the chops are. Thick pork chops need a longer cooking time. It's okay, though, for the lamb to be a little pink on the inside. Serve with lemon wedges and herb butter.

Nutritional value (per serving):

Net Carbohydrates: 0% (0.3 g)

Fiber: 0 g

Fat: 76% (62 g)

Protein: 23% (43 g)

kcal: 723

56. Zesty Chili Lime Keto Tuna Salad

Preparation time: 5 minutes Cooking time: none
Total time: 5 minutes Yield: 1 cup

Ingredients

1/3 cup of mayonnaise

1 tablespoon of lime juice 1/4 teaspoon of salt
1/8 teaspoon of pepper
1 teaspoon Tajin chili lime seasoning 1 medium celery (finely chopped)
2 tablespoons red onion (finely chopped) 2 cups romaine lettuce (roughly chopped) 5 oz canned tuna
Optional: chopped green onion, black pepper, lemon juice

Instructions

Add mayonnaise, lime juice, salt, pepper, and chili lime spices to a medium bowl. Stir well until smooth. Add vegetables and tuna to the bowl and stir to coat. Serve with celery, cucumber, or on a bed of vegetables.

Nutritional value (per serving):

Serving Size: ½ cup Calories: 406
Fat: 37 g
Carbohydrates: Net Carbohydrates: 1 g

Preparation time: 5 minutes Cooking time: 15 minutes Total time: 20 minutes Yield: 5

Ingredients

1 pound organic ground turkey (or ground beef, lamb, or pork) 2 cups of seasoned cauliflower

2 tablespoons coconut oil

1/2 a Vidalia onion 2 cloves of garlic

2 cups of full-fat coconut milk (or heavy cream) 1 tbsp. mustard

1 teaspoon: salt, black pepper, thyme, celery salt, garlic powder

Instructions

Heat the coconut oil in a large pan. Meanwhile, finely chop the onion and garlic. Add it to the hot oil. Stir for 2-3 minutes and then add the ground turkey. Spread with the spatula and stir constantly until crumbled.

Add the spice mix and the sliced cauliflower and stir well. When the meat is brown, add the coconut milk, bring to the boil and reduce for 5-8 minutes, stirring regularly. At this point, it is ready to serve. Or you can reduce it by half until thick and serve as a dip. Mix in grated cheese for an extra thick sauce.

Nutritional value (per serving):

Calories: 388

Fat: 30.5

Carbohydrates: 5.5

Protein: 28.8

Preparation time: 10 minutes Cooking time: 40 minutes Total time: 50 minutes Yield: 5

Ingredients
5 small chicken breasts or chicken breast cutlets 1 cup of savoy cabbage
5 slices of prosciutto
3 tablespoons coconut flour 2 tsp salt, more to taste
1 tsp black pepper
2 tsp Italian spice mix 1/2 cup of bone broth 1/4 cup avocado oil

Instructions
Preheat the oven to 400F. Combine the chicken breast, salt, pepper, herbs, and coconut flour in a gallon-sized plastic bag. Shake to evenly coat the chicken, yes, like shake and bake!
Sprinkle a tablespoon. of the oil on the baking tray.

Chop the savoy cabbage and make 5 small stacks of grated cabbage on the baking tray. Sprinkle with a little salt. Drizzle a little oil over it. Top with a coated chicken fillet. Finally, cover each piece of chicken with a slice of prosciutto. Drizzle with the remaining oil.

Roast at 400F for 30 minutes. Pour the stock into the baking pan. Roast for another 10 minutes. Remove from oven and serve warm. Use a spatula to scoop up one pile at a time.

Nutritional value (per serving):
Calories: 369
Fat: 24.8
Carbohydrates: 5.8
Protein: 33.7

Preparation time: 15 minutes Cooking time: 15 minutes Total time: 30 minutes Yield: 5

Ingredients
1 pound skirt steak
3 tablespoons coconut oil
2 tablespoons coconut Aminos 1 tbsp. apple cider vinegar
1 tsp garlic powder 1 tsp ginger powder 1 teaspoon of salt
1 tsp coconut flour

Instructions
Tender your steak with a kitchen mallet (or heavy-bottomed pan). That's right, save your steak. Then cut it into thin strips. Toss in a bowl with coconut Aminos and apple cider vinegar. Marinate for 10 minutes.

Heat a wok or large cast-iron skillet. When it comes to temperature, use tongs to put the strips of steak in the wok. Cooking in batches so that the meat browns quickly, 3-4 minutes per batch, would take about 3 batches. When all the strips are brown, put them back in the wok and mix with the coconut flour. Then add the vinegar and coconut Amino from the marinating bowl and fry for a few minutes until the meat is glazed with a brown sauce. If you're making cauliflower rice, cook it in the same hot wok! Serve your bowl, garnish, and dig in!

Nutritional value (per serving):
Calories: 242
Fat: 18
Saturated fat: 18
Carbohydrates: 3
Protein: 24.9

60. Keto Fried Chicken

Preparation time: 15 minutes Cooking time: 40 minutes Total time: 55 minutes Yield: 6 pcs

Ingredients
6 boneless chicken thighs 4 oz ground pork rinds
2 tsp ground thyme 2 tsp salt
1 ½ tsp paprika powder
1 tsp garlic powder or 1 tbsp. crushed fresh garlic
¼ tsp ground cayenne pepper
¼ tsp black pepper
1 egg
¼ cup of mayonnaise 2 tbsp hot sauce
1 tbsp mustard

Instructions
Preheat the oven to 425 ° F and line the baking sheet with parchment paper or aluminum foil and place the baking rack on top. Pat each piece of chicken dry with kitchen paper. Put aside. Combine dry ingredients in a small mixing bowl. Beat together until completely absorbed. Transfer half of the dry ingredients into a shallow bowl. In a separate bowl, combine egg, mayonnaise, hot sauce, and mustard.

Dip the chicken pieces one at a time in the egg wash and then in dry ingredients, turning them over several times to completely cover the chicken with the dry breading mixture. Place the breaded chicken on the baking rack on a baking tray. Continue to bread the remaining chicken thighs. Bake until internal temperature reaches 165 ° F, about 35-40 minutes, depending on the thickness of the chicken thigh. Let them cool slightly before serving.

Nutritional value (per serving):

Serving Size: 1 piece

Calories: 372

Fat: 23 g

Carbohydrates: 0.9 g (0.6 g net)

Protein: 41.2 g

61. Grilled lamb liver

10 minutes preparation
45 minutes of cooking time Portions 2

Ingredients

100 g lamb liver
½ cup of sliced kale
2 tablespoons of butter 1 tablespoon of olive oil
½ teaspoon of dried rosemary
½ teaspoons freshly ground black pepper 2 tablespoons of lime juice
Salt

Instructions

Prepare the marinade by mixing the butter, lime juice, black pepper, olive oil, and rosemary in a bowl. Add the liver and finely chopped kale to the bowl and marinate for 10-15 minutes. Preheat the grill pan on the stove and add the liver. Cook for 2-3 minutes on each side. Remove the grill pan from the heat and add the chopped kale. Toss and turn to mix well with the butter, rosemary, and lamb liver juice.

Nutritional value

Net carbs: 2% (5 g)
Fiber: 1 g
Fats: 82% (79 g)
Protein: 16% (34 g)
kcal: 875

10 minutes preparation
50 minutes of cooking time Portions 6

Ingredients
75 g chicken
1 clove of garlic
½ cup of bamboo shoots 1 tablespoon of butter
1 tablespoon of olive oil 1 dried red chili
Chives
Salt and pepper

Instructions
Heat olive oil in a frying pan. Add the garlic and cook until it turns brown. Add the dried red chili and bamboo shoots and cook for about 3 minutes. Add the chicken, salt, and pepper. Stir and cook until the chicken is about 7 minutes. Toss in the chives and cook for 2 more minutes. Add the butter and let it sizzle for 1 minute. Place the chicken and bamboo shoots.

Nutritional value
Net carbs: 2% (5 g)
Fiber: 1 g
Fats: 82% (79 g)
Protein: 16% (34 g)
kcal: 875

63. Crab And Zucchini Casserole

5 minutes preparation 45 minutes cooking time Portions 4

Ingredients
100 g crab meat
½ cup of sliced zucchini 4 asparagus
1 teaspoon of olive oil
1 sprig of fresh rosemary
½ cup of shredded cheddar cheese 1 clove of crushed garlic
Salt and pepper

Instructions
Blanch the zucchini and asparagus in a cooking pot. Add olive oil, rosemary, and garlic in a skillet. Fry until the garlic turns brown. Add the crabmeat, salt, and pepper. Cook for about 2 minutes. In an oven dish, first, add the zucchini and then a layer of crab meat. Then put the asparagus on top. Add the grated cheddar cheese to the asparagus and bake at 180 degrees C for 20-30 minutes.

Nutritional value
Net carbs: 3% (5 g)
Fiber: 1 g
Fat: 75% (52 g)
Protein: 21% (33 g)
kcal: 625

10 minutes preparation

15 minutes of cooking time Portions 6

Ingredients

100 g salmon fillet

½ cup of broccoli

2 teaspoons of butter

½ teaspoon of dried rosemary

½ teaspoon of dried thyme

½ teaspoon of garlic oil

2 tablespoons of mayonnaise with chili oil Salt and pepper

Instructions

Mix 1 dried rosemary, dried thyme, 1 teaspoon of butter, garlic oil, salt, and pepper in a bowl. Rub it over the salmon fillet. Preheat the grill and grill the salmon and broccoli for 6-7 minutes. Add 1 teaspoon of butter to the salmon. Sprinkle the broccoli with salt and pepper. Serve the grilled salmon and broccoli with mayonnaise-chili oil dip.

Nutritional value

Net Carbohydrates: 2% (1 g)

Fiber: 0 g

Fat: 71% (16 g)

Protein: 27% (13 g)

kcal: 205

5 minutes preparation

20 minutes of cooking time Portions 4

Ingredients

1 cup of spinach 2 eggs

¼ cup of finely chopped celery

½ teaspoon of garlic paste 2 teaspoons of butter

2 tablespoons of grated cheddar cheese 1 teaspoon of dried oregano

Salt and pepper

Instructions

Add a pinch of salt and pepper to the eggs and beat together. Place a skillet over medium heat. Pour 1 teaspoon of butter and let the butter melt. Add the garlic paste and cook for 30 seconds. Add the spinach, celery, salt, and pepper. Cook for about 30 seconds. Remove the spinach and celery from the skillet and add 1 teaspoon of butter. Add the beaten eggs and cook like an omelet for 2 minutes over medium heat. Add the baked spinach and cheddar cheese. Sprinkle with oregano and wrap the omelet around the spinach, celery, and cheddar filling. Let it cook until the cheese melts. Eat while it is still warm.

Nutritional value

Net Carbohydrates: 2% (1 g)

Fiber: 0 g

Fat: 71% (16 g)

Protein: 27% (13 g)

kcal: 205

Dinner

66. Keto zucchini rolls with chicken and herb butter

15 minutes of preparation 40 minutes of cooking time Portions 4

Ingredients
Zucchini roll-ups
1½ pounds of zucchini
½ tsp salt 3 oz. butter
6 oz. mushrooms, finely chopped 6 oz. cream cheese
6 oz. grated cheese
1 green pepper, finely chopped
2 ounces air-dried chorizo, finely chopped 1 egg
1 tsp onion powder
2 tbsp fresh parsley, chopped
½ tsp salt
¼ teaspoon of pepper Chicken
4 chicken breasts, with bone and skin (about 180 grams each) Salt and pepper
1 oz. butter, for baking Herb butter
4 oz. butter, at room temperature 1 clove of garlic, chopped
1 tbsp fresh parsley, finely chopped 1 teaspoon of lemon juice
½ tsp salt

Instructions
Preheat the oven to 350 ° F (175 ° C). Cut the zucchini lengthwise into half-centimeter slices and place on a baking tray lined with parchment paper. Season with salt and let stand for ten minutes. Dry the liquid with kitchen paper. Baking in the oven for 20 minutes, until the zucchini is soft. Remove from the oven and let cool on wire rack. If necessary, dry off some more liquid.

Heat a large frying pan with butter and brown the mushrooms. Let cool. Add all other ingredients, except a third of the grated cheese, to a bowl. Add mushrooms and mix well. Place a generous amount of cheese batter on each zucchini slice. Roll up and place the roll- ups seam down in an oven dish. Sprinkle with the rest of the cheese.

Increase the temperature to 400 ° F (200 ° C). Bake for 20 minutes or until the cheese has some color. Meanwhile, season the chicken and fry in butter over medium heat until golden and cooked through.

Herb butter

Mix all ingredients thoroughly in a small bowl. Serve with the chicken rolls.

Nutritional value

Net carbs: 4% (10 g)
Fiber: 3 g
Fat: 80% (82 g)
Protein: 15% (35 g)
kcal: 913

15 minutes preparation 20 minutes cooking time Portions 2

Ingredients
Pimiento cheese
1/3 cup of mayonnaise
¼ cup of pimientos or pickled jalapeños 1 tsp paprika or chili powder
1 tbsp Dijon mustard
1 pinch of cayenne pepper 4 oz. cheddar cheese, grated Meatballs
1½ pounds ground beef 1 egg
Salt and pepper
2 tbsp butter, for frying

Instructions
Start by mixing all the ingredients for the pimiento cheese in a large bowl. Add ground beef and egg to the cheese mixture. Use a wooden spoon or clean hands to combine. Salt and Pepper to taste. Form large meatballs and fry them in butter or oil in a skillet over medium heat until well cooked. Serve with a side dish of your choice, a green salad, and possibly a homemade mayonnaise.

Nutritional value
Net Carbohydrates: 1% (1 g)
Fiber: 1 g
Fats: 73% (52 g)
Protein: 26% (41 g)
kcal: 651

15 minutes preparation
40 minutes of cooking time Portions 4

Ingredients
Pork chops
2 tbsp mild chipotle paste 2 tbsp olive oil
½ tsp salt
1¾ lbs pork shoulder chops (4 chops) Garlic butter topping
4 oz. butter, at room temperature 1 clove of garlic
½ tsp salt
¼ tsp ground black pepper
¼ tsp paprika powder Green beans and avocado 2 tbsp olive oil
2/3 pound of fresh green beans
½ tsp salt
¼ tsp ground black pepper 2 avocados
6 spring onions
Fresh cilantro (optional) Pepper to taste

Instructions
In a small bowl, combine chipotle paste, oil, and salt. Brush the meat with the marinade and let it rest for 15 minutes. You can also marinate the meat in a plastic bag in the refrigerator for 30 minutes or more.

Preheat the oven to 400 ° F (200 ° C). Grill the marinated meat on a wire rack on a baking tray in the oven for 20-30 minutes until the meat is cooked. Turn over after 10-15 minutes. Meanwhile, make the herb butter. Crush the garlic clove, mix with butter and herbs, and set aside. Heat the oil in a frying pan. Fry the beans over medium heat for about 5 minutes until they have a nice color.

Lower the heat towards the end and add spices. Finely chop the onion. Peel and stone the avocado and coarsely mash the flesh with a fork. Stir the onion and avocado into the beans. Season with Salt and Pepper. Finish with a handful of finely chopped cilantro.

Nutritional value
Net carbs: 3% (6 g)
Fiber: 9 g
Fats: 79% (76 g)
Protein: 18% (38 g)
kcal: 883

10 minutes preparation
10 minutes of cooking time Portions 2

Ingredients
½ cup of mayonnaise 2 tbsp Dijon mustard 1 shallot
1 pickle with dill 4 oz. lettuce
8 oz. pastrami
4 eggs
4 low- carb parmesan croutons

Instructions
Start making the low- carb parmesan croutons, if you don't already have them on hand. Stir together mayonnaise and mustard and set aside. Divide the lettuce between two plates. Chop the onion and put it on top. Cut the pickled cucumber into four pieces lengthwise and place it on top of the lettuce. Add pastrami and a generous amount of mustard mayonnaise. Fry the eggs just before serving the salad. Sunnyside up or easy, and serve right away with parmesan croutons.

Nutritional value
Net carbs: 3% (5 g)
Fiber: 2 g
Fat: 75% (57 g)
Protein: 22% (38 g)
kcal: 696

5 minutes preparation 45 minutes cooking time Portions 4

Ingredients
½ cup of almond flour 4 tbsp coconut flour

½ tsp salt

1 tsp baking powder 2½ oz. butter

6 oz. grated cheese

1 egg

1 pound link sausages or uncured hot dogs 1 egg, to brush the dough

16 cloves, for the eyes of the mummy (optional)

Instructions
Preheat the oven to 350 ° F (175 ° C). In a large bowl, combine almond flour, coconut flour, and baking powder. Melt the butter and cheese in a pan over low heat. Stir well with a wooden spoon for a smooth and flexible batter. Remove from heat after a few minutes. Stir the egg into the flour mixture and then add the cheese mixture into a firm dough.

Make a rectangle about 8 × 14 inches (20 × 35 cm). Cut into 8 long strips, less than an inch wide (1.5-2 cm). Wrap the dough strips around the hot dog and brush with a beaten egg. Place on a baking tray lined with parchment paper and bake for 15-20 minutes until the dough is golden brown. The hot dog is then also ready. Push two cloves into each hot dog to make them look like eyes - but only for decoration. Don't eat the cloves!

Nutritional value
Net Carbs: 4% (7 g)

Fiber: 4 g

Fats: 81% (67 g)

Protein: 15% (29 g)

kcal: 759

15 minutes preparation
30 minutes of cooking time Portions 4

Ingredients
Pie crust
1 cup of almond flour 4½ tbsp sesame seeds 1/3 cup of coconut flour
1 tbsp ground psyllium husk powder 1 tsp baking powder
½ tsp salt
1 egg
¼ cup of water
2 tbsp light olive oil

Stuffing
10 oz. mushrooms, chanterelles 2 ounces butter, for baking
1 tsp dried thyme Salt and pepper
4 eggs
11/3 cups of heavy whipping cream 5 oz. Parmesan cheese

Instructions
Preheat the oven to 365 ° F (185 ° C). Mix all ingredients for the pie crust in a food processor for 1-2 minutes, until you get a firm dough. If you don't have a food processor, simply knead the ingredients together in a bowl with a fork or your hands. Let rest in the refrigerator for 5-10 minutes.

Roll out the dough, about 1/4-inch (1/2 cm) thick, between two sheets of parchment paper. You can also use well-oiled hands or a spatula to spread the dough directly into a non-stick cake pan. If you use tin, place parchment paper between the ring and the bottom to the baked cake easier separately to make.

Clean the mushrooms and fry them in butter until golden brown. Add thyme, salt, and pepper to taste. Beat the rest of the ingredients together and pour into the pie crust. Add mushrooms. Keep some nice ones for decoration/serving. Bake for 30 minutes or until the cake turns a nice golden brown color and the filling is firm. Let cool for a few minutes before serving.

Nutritional value
Net Carbohydrates: 4% (9 g)
Fiber: 9 g
Fats: 82% (84 g)
Protein: 14% (33 g)
kcal: 938

25 minutes preparation
15 minutes of cooking time Portions 10

Ingredients
½ cup of almond flour
¼ cup of coconut flour
½ tsp salt
1 tsp baking powder 1 egg, beaten
2 ounces butter
6½ oz. grated cheese, preferably mozzarella
¼ cup of green pesto
1 egg, beaten to coat the top

Instructions
Preheat the oven to 350 ° F (175 ° C). Mix all dry ingredients in a bowl. Add the egg and mix. Melt the butter and cheese together in a pan over low heat. Stir until the batter is smooth. Slowly add the butter cheese batter to the dry mixing bowl and mix into a stiff dough.

Place the dough on parchment paper the size of a rectangular baking tray. Using a rolling pin, make a rectangle about 1/5-inch (5mm) thick. Divide the pesto over it and cut it into 2.5 cm strips. Turn them over and place them on a baking tray lined with parchment paper. Brush twists with the beaten egg. Bake in the oven for 15-20 minutes until golden brown.

Nutritional value
Net Carbohydrates: 3% (1 g)
Fiber: 2 g
Fats: 81% (17 g)
Protein: 16% (8 g)
kcal: 194

73. Keto Caprese omelet

10 minutes preparation 10 minutes cooking time Portions 2

Ingredients
6 eggs
Salt and pepper
1 tbsp chopped fresh basil or dried basil 2 tbsp olive oil
3 oz. cherry tomatoes halved or tomatoes cut into slices 5 oz. fresh mozzarella cheese, diced or sliced

Instructions
Crack the eggs in a mixing bowl; add salt and black pepper to taste. Beat well with a fork until completely combined. Add basil and stir. Heat the oil in a large frying pan. Fry the tomatoes for a few minutes. Pour the egg batter over the tomatoes. Wait for the batter to set before adding the mozzarella cheese. Lower the heat and let the omelet solidify. Serve immediately and enjoy!

Nutritional value
Net carbs: 3% (4 g)
Fiber: 1 g
Fats: 72% (43 g)
Protein: 25% (33 g)
kcal: 534

74. Keto fried bacon omelet

5 minutes preparation 20 minutes cooking time Portions 2

Ingredients
4 eggs
5 oz. bacon cut into cubes 3 oz. butter
2 ounces fresh spinach
1 tablespoon finely chopped fresh chives (optional) Salt and pepper

Instructions
Preheat the oven to 400 ° F (200 ° C). Grease an individual baking dish with butter. Fry bacon and spinach in the remaining butter. Beat the eggs until frothy. Mix in the spinach and bacon, including the fat leftover from frying. Add some finely chopped chives. Season with Salt and Pepper. Pour the egg mixture into the baking dish (s) and bake for 20 minutes or until firm and golden brown. Let cool for a few minutes and serve.

Nutritional value
Net Carbohydrates: 1% (2 g)
Fiber: 1 g
Fat: 87% (72 g)
Protein: 12% (21 g)
kcal: 737

75. Keto chicken wings with creamy broccoli

10 minutes preparation 45 minutes of cooking time Portions 2

Ingredients
Fried chicken wings
½ orange, juice, and zest
¼ cup of olive oil
2 tsp ginger powder 1 teaspoon of salt
¼ tsp cayenne pepper 3 lbs chicken wings
Creamy broccoli
1½ pounds of broccoli 1 cup of mayonnaise
¼ cup of chopped fresh dill Salt and pepper, to taste

Instructions
Preheat the oven to 400 ° F (200 ° C). In a small bowl, mix juice and zest of the orange with oil and spices. Place the chicken wings in a plastic bag and add the marinade. Shake the bag well to cover the wings well. Set aside to marinate for at least 5 minutes, but preferably longer. Place the wings in one layer in a greased baking dish or on a grill rack for extra crunchiness.

Bake on the middle rack in the oven for about 45 minutes or until the wings are golden and well cooked. In the meantime, divide the broccoli into small florets and boil them in salted water for a few minutes. They should only soften a little but do not lose their shape or color. Strain the broccoli and let some of the steam evaporate before adding the remaining ingredients. Serve the broccoli with the fried wings.

Nutritional value
Net Carbs: 3% (9 g)
Fiber: 5 g
Fat: 75% (100 g)
Protein: 22% (65 g)
kcal: 1216

76. Keto crab meat and egg plate

5 minutes preparation
10 minutes of cooking time Portions 2

Ingredients
4 eggs
12 oz. canned crabmeat 2 avocados
½ cup of cottage cheese
½ cup of mayonnaise 1½ oz. baby spinach 2 tbsp olive oil
½ tsp chili flakes (optional) Salt and pepper

Instructions
Start cooking the eggs. Gently lower them into boiling water and let them cook for 4-8 minutes, depending on whether you want them soft or hard-boiled. Chill the eggs in ice-cold water for 1-2 minutes when cooked; this makes it easier to remove the shell. Peel the eggs. Place the eggs, crab, avocado, curd cheese, mayonnaise and spinach on a plate. Drizzle olive oil over the spinach. Season with salt and pepper. Sprinkle optional chili flakes over the avocado and serve.

Nutritional value
Net carbs: 3% (7 g)
Fiber: 14 g
Fat: 81% (96 g)
Protein: 16% (43 g)
kcal: 1100

Serve for 4 people
Time in total: 19 minutes

Ingredients:
½ tsp coconut butter
1 medium diced onion 450-500 g chicken fillet 1 chopped garlic
Two medium-sized courgettes 400 g of crushed tomatoes
7-10 cherry tomatoes (half cut)
100 g raw cashew nuts * (for spices: turmeric, paprika, and salt) For
herbs: salt, pepper, dry oregano & basil

Instructions:
Heat a large pan over medium/high heat. Add coconut butter and
diced onions. Cook for 30 seconds to 1 minute. Be careful not to
burn the onions. Cut the chicken into 2 cm pieces. Add chicken
and chopped garlic to a pan. Season with basil, oregano salt, and
pepper. Fry the chicken for 5-6 minutes or until golden brown.

While the chicken is cooking, spiral the zucchini. Cut them shorter
if necessary. If you don't have a special spiralizer, just use your
vegetable peeler and make zucchini ribbons. Add crushed
tomatoes and simmer for 3-5 minutes. Roast the cashews in
another pan (or oven) until golden brown. Season with paprika,
turmeric, and salt. Finally add spiral Zoodles, cherry tomatoes, and
season with additional salt if needed. Cook for 1 more minute and
then turn off the heat. Serve the chicken zoodles with spiced
cashews and fresh basil. To enjoy!

Nutritional value (per serving):
 411, 1 kcal
Proteins: 45.7 g
Net carbs: 11.7 g
Fat: 18.8 g

Prep Time 10 Minutes
Cooking Time 15 Minutes
Total Time 25 Minutes
6 servings

Ingredients
1.25 pounds skinless chicken breasts, thinly sliced
1.67 tablespoons of olive oil
0.83 cup of heavy cream
0.42 cup of chicken stock
0.83 teaspoon of garlic powder
0.83 teaspoon of Italian herbs
0.42 cup of parmesan cheese
0.83 cup spinach chopped
0.42 cup of sun-dried tomatoes

Instructions
Add in a large frying pan olive oil and fry the chicken over medium heat for 3-5 minutes on each side or until browned on each side and cook until no longer pink in the middle. Remove the chicken and set aside on a plate.

Add the whipped cream, chicken stock, garlic powder, Italian herbs, and Parmesan cheese. Beat over medium heat until it starts to thicken. Add the spinach and sun-dried tomatoes and let it simmer until the spinach starts to wilt. Add the chicken back to the pan and serve over pasta if desired.

Nutritional value
Fat 25g38%
Saturated fat 12 g 60%
Cholesterol 133 mg 44%
Sodium 379 mg 16%

(2-3 servings)

Ingredients:
2 limes
1 red pepper, seeded and julienned
1/2 green bell pepper, seeded and julienned 1/2 large yellow onion, thinly sliced
2 teaspoons plus 1/3 cup of canola oil, divided 2 cloves of garlic
1 teaspoon of kosher salt
1/2 teaspoon of dried oregano 1/2 teaspoon chili powder
1/2 teaspoon of sweet paprika 1/2 teaspoon of cayenne pepper 1/4 teaspoon of cumin powder
1 pound (41/50 measure) raw shrimp, gutted and peeled 6 flour tortillas
Mexican crema, sour cream or Greek yogurt

Instructions:
Preheat the oven to 400 ° F. Place the baking pan close by.
Squeeze 1 1/2 of the limes. Cut the other half of the lime into six wedges and set them aside. Toss the bell pepper and onion in the 2 teaspoons of canola oil until covered. Divide them in a single layer over the baking tray. Pour the lime juice and garlic into a blender and add the remaining oil in a steady stream. Add the salt and spices, pulsing once to combine. Marinate the shrimp and stir in a large zip-top bag for 15 minutes

In the meantime, roast the bell pepper and onion for 10 minutes. Remove the shrimp from the marinade. Polka dot the shrimp on the baking sheet with roasted vegetables. Roast for another 8 minutes or until pink and fragrant. Heat some flour tortillas and put down the Mexican crema or sour cream to serve with the lime wedges.

Prep Time: 20 Minutes Cooking Time: 15 Minutes Total Time: 20 Minutes Yield: 4 Services

Ingredients

1 teaspoon of salt, divided
1 pound turkey fillet, cut into thin steaks of about ¼ inch thick sliced
2 tablespoons of extra virgin olive oil, divided
½ large sweet onion, sliced 1 red pepper, cut into strips
1 yellow pepper, cut into strips
½ teaspoon of Italian herbs
¼ teaspoon ground black pepper 2 teaspoons of red wine vinegar
1 14-ounce can tomatoes, preferably fire-roasted Chopped fresh parsley and basil for garnish (optional)

Instructions

Sprinkle ½ teaspoon of salt over turkey. Heat 1 tablespoon of oil in a large non-stick frying pan over medium heat. Add half of the turkey and cook, until brown on the bottom, 1 to 3 minutes. Flip and continue to cook until completely cooked 1 to 2 minutes. Place the turkey on a plate with a slotted spatula, tent with foil to keep warm. Add the remaining 1 tablespoon of oil to the pan, reduce the heat to medium and repeat with the remaining turkey, 1 to 3 minutes per side.

Add onion, bell pepper, and remaining ½ teaspoon of salt to the pan, cover, and cook, removing the lid to stir often until onion and bell pepper turn soft and blotchy brown, 5 to 7 minutes. Remove lid, increase heat to medium-low, drizzle with Italian herbs and pepper and cook, stirring often, until spices are fragrant, about 30 seconds. Add vinegar and cook, stirring until almost completely evaporated, about 20 seconds. Add tomatoes and bring to a boil, stirring frequently.

Add the turkey to the pan with any accumulated juices from the plate and bring it to a boil. Reduce heat to medium-low and cook, turning sauce over until turkey is completely hot, 1 to 2 minutes. Serve with parsley and basil if desired.

Nutritional values per serving
Calories: 230 Calories
Sugar: 7 g
Sodium: 635 Mg
Fat: 8 g
Saturated Fat: 1 g
Carbohydrates: 11 g
Fiber: 3 g
Protein: 30g

Cooking time: 20 minutes Preparation time: 10 minutes Cooking time: 20 minutes Servings: 6

Ingredients
1.5 lbs of chicken breast cut into cubes 2 tablespoons of garam masala

3 teaspoons fresh ginger grated 3 teaspoons of minced garlic

4 oz whole milk Greek yogurt 1 tablespoon of coconut oil

Sauce:
2 tablespoons of ghee or butter 1 onion

2 teaspoons of fresh ginger grated 2 teaspoons of chopped garlic

14.5 oz can have crushed tomatoes 1 tablespoon of ground coriander

½ tablespoon of garam masala 2 teaspoons of cumin

1 teaspoon chili powder

½ cup of whipped cream Salt to taste

Optional for serving:

Chopped cilantro Cauliflower rice Sliced fresh jalapeños

Instructions
Cut the chicken into 5 cm pieces and place in a large bowl with 2 tablespoons of garam masala, 1 teaspoon of grated ginger, and 1 teaspoon of chopped garlic. Add the yogurt, stir to combine. Transfer to the refrigerator and refrigerate for at least 30 minutes.

For the sauce, put the onion, ginger, garlic, crushed tomatoes, and herbs in a blender and blend until smooth. Put aside. Heat 1 tablespoon of oil in a large skillet over medium heat. Place the chicken in the pan along with the marinade and brown for 3 to 4 minutes per side. Once browned, pour the sauce and cook for 5 to 6 minutes longer.

Stir in the whipped cream and ghee and cook for another minute. Taste for salt and add extra if necessary. Finish with cilantro and serve with cauliflower rice if desired.

Nutritional values per serving
Fats 17g26%
Saturated fat 10 g 63%
Cholesterol 111 mg 37%
Sodium 278 mg 12%
Potassium 724 mg

82. Keto crab meat and egg plate

5 minutes preparation
10 minutes of cooking time Portions 2

Ingredients
4 eggs
12 oz. canned crabmeat 2 avocados
½ cup of cottage cheese
½ cup of mayonnaise 1½ oz. baby spinach 2 tbsp olive oil
½ tsp chili flakes (optional) Salt and pepper

Instructions
Start cooking the eggs. Gently lower them into boiling water and let them cook for 4-8 minutes, depending on whether you want them soft or hard-boiled. Chill the eggs in ice-cold water for 1-2 minutes when cooked; this makes it easier to remove the shell. Peel the eggs. Place the eggs, crab, avocado, curd cheese, mayonnaise and spinach on a plate. Drizzle olive oil over the spinach. Season with salt and pepper. Sprinkle optional chili flakes over the avocado and serve.

Nutritional value
Net carbs: 3% (7 g)
Fiber: 14 g
Fat: 81% (96 g)
Protein: 16% (43 g)
kcal: 1100

Preparation time: 10 minutes Cooking time: 20 minutes

Ingredients

3 chicken breasts

1 teaspoon of garlic paste

12 Asparagus stems removed 1/2 cup of cream cheese

1 tablespoon of butter 1 teaspoon Olive oil 3/4 cup marinara sauce

1 cup of mozzarella shredded Salt and pepper to taste

Instructions

To start cooking the chicken, butterfly the chicken (or cut it in half without cutting it all the way through. The chicken breast should open like a butterfly with one end intact in the center). Remove the hardy stems from the asparagus and set aside.

Rub salt, pepper, and garlic paste over the chicken breasts (inside and out). Divide the cream cheese over the chicken fillets and spread it on the inside. Place four stalks of asparagus and fold one side of the breast over the other, tucking it in place with a toothpick to keep it from opening.

Preheat the oven and put it on the grill. Add butter and olive oil to a hot skillet and place the chicken breasts in it. Cook the breasts on each side for 6-7 minutes (total time is 14-15 minutes depending on the size of the breast) until the chicken is almost cooked.

Cover each breast with 1/4 cup of marinara sauce and spread the grated mozzarella on top. Place in the oven and roast for 5 minutes until the cheese melts.

Nutritional values

Calories: 572kcal

Carbohydrates: 10g

Protein: 62g

Fat: 31 g Saturated fat: 14 g

Cholesterol: 216 mg

Preparation time: 5 minutes Cooking time: 25 minutes Total time: 30 minutes Servings: 6 servings

Ingredients

4 chicken fillets large cut into pieces 1 tbsp butter

½ onions chopped

2 cups of chicken stock

10 oz canned diced tomatoes, undrained 2 oz tomato paste

1 tbsp chili powder 1 tbsp cumin

1/2 tbsp garlic powder

1 chopped jalapeno pepper (optional) 4 oz cream cheese

Salt and pepper to taste

Instructions

Prepare the chicken by boiling chicken breasts in water or stock on a stovetop for 10-12 minutes, just below the liquid. Once the meat is no longer pink, remove it from the liquid and cut with two forks. The same technique can also be used with a pressure cooker under pressure for 5 minutes with a natural release, or a slow cooker for 4-6 hours. Whatever is smart for you! Rotisserie chicken meat can also be substituted for the breasts.

Melt the butter in a large stockpot over medium heat. Add the onion and cook until translucent. Add the shredded chicken, chicken stock, diced tomatoes, tomato puree, chili powder, cumin, garlic powder, and jalapeno to the pan and mix by gently stirring over the burner. Bring to a boil, then simmer over medium heat and cover for 10 minutes. Cut cream cheese into small 2.5 cm pieces.

Remove the lid and mix in the cream cheese. Increase the heat back to medium and keep stirring until the cream cheese is completely mixed. Remove from heat and season with salt and pepper. Eat as is or garnish with toppings of your choice. I like cilantro and Monterey Jack cheese for ooey-gooey goodness.

Nutritional values
Calories: 201kcal
Carbohydrates: 7g
Protein: 18g
Fat: 11 g Saturated fat: 5 g
Cholesterol: 74 mg

Servings: 6
Preparation time: 5 minutes Cooking time: 15 minutes

Ingredients
1 pound ground beef 1 tbsp chili powder
½ teaspoon of salt
¾ teaspoon of cumin
½ teaspoon of dried oregano
¼ teaspoon of garlic powder
¼ teaspoon of onion powder 4 ounces of tomato sauce
3 avocados cut in half
1 cup of cheddar cheese, shredded
¼ cup cherry tomatoes, chopped
¼ cup of lettuce, cut into pieces

Additional toppings:
Coriander Sour cream

Instructions
Add the ground beef to a medium saucepan. Cook over medium heat until brown. Drain the fat and add the herbs and tomato sauce. Stir to combine. Cook for about 3-4 minutes. Remove the stone from the halved avocados. Load the crater to the left of the pit with the taco meat. Top with cheese, tomatoes, lettuce, cilantro, and sour cream. If you want a larger portion of avocado for the toppings, then spoon some of the avocados and set aside guacamole make ! Then fill with toppings.

Nutritional values
1g, calories: 410kcal
Protein: 26g
cholesterol: 70mg

86. Bowls of beef and broccoli with sun sauce

Preparation time: 10
Total time: 30
Yield: 4 bowls

Ingredients

For the beef
1 tablespoon of shortening
1 pound 85% lean grass-fed ground beef 1 teaspoon of fine salt
1 teaspoon of garlic powder
1 tablespoon of coconut Aminos

For the broccoli
4 broccoli crowns cut into florets 1 tablespoon of avocado oil
1/2 teaspoon of fine salt

For the sun sauce
1 tablespoon of shortening
2 tablespoons of sunflower seed or cashew butter 1/4 cup of bone broth
1 teaspoon of ginger powder 1/2 fine salt
2 teaspoons of coconut Aminos juice of a lemon
1 green onion, finely chopped

Collect
4 cups of baby spinach (optional)

Instructions
Preheat the oven to 400F. Toss the broccoli with fat and salt to massage a sheet pan of the fat in the florets, they spread them out over the baking tray, so that they are not crowded. Set the baking pan while it is preheating, once it comes to temperature,

set a time for 20 minutes. Meanwhile, heat a large skillet over medium heat, adding the fat for temperature.

Crumble the ground beef in the pan and add the salt and garlic. Stir; break it with a whisk until brown and crumbly. Add the coconut Aminos and bring the heat to high. Cook and keep stirring occasionally, until dark brown and crispy. While that cook is setting, put a small saucepan over medium heat. Melt the fat and then the sunflower seed butter, stirring until smooth.

Add the bone stock, salt, amino, and ground ginger stir until well blended and dark brown. Remove from heat and stir in lemon juice and stir until smooth again. Mix in the green onion. Put aside. To assemble the bowls, make a bed of baby spinach in 4 large bowls. Spoon ground beef into each of the bowls. Add the broccoli florets and spoon the sauce over everything. Dig in!

Nutritional values
Press size: 1 bowl
Calories: 388
Fat: 29 g
Carbohydrates: 14 g
Fiber: 8 g
Protein: 30 g

Ingredients

1/2 cup of medium cauliflower 2 large eggs

2 cloves of garlic chopped 100 g pork belly

2 mini green peppers 2 spring onions

1 tablespoon of soy sauce or tamari 1 teaspoon of black sesame seeds

1 tsp pickled ginger

Instructions

Prepare the flour. Cut the cauliflower into florets. Place in a food processor and pulse until rice grains form. Don't go too far or you'll end up with cauliflower puree instead! Heat some oil in a frying pan (or wok), add the cauliflower and fry over medium heat for about 5 minutes. Remove from pan and set aside. Prepare the fried rice.

Then make your omelet with eggs loose to beat and add to your skillet. Stir the mixture to make a thin omelet. When it is cooked, turn and cook for another minute. Remove from pan and set aside. Add your garlic to the skillet and once it is fragrant add the pork belly. Cut your omelet into small cubes while cooking.

When the pork belly is cooked, add the bell pepper, half of the spring onion and cook for another minute. Then add the cauliflower and egg back to the pan. Add the soy sauce and stir well. Cook over high heat until well combined and serve to steam hot. Garnish with the remaining spring onions, sesame seeds, and pickled ginger. To enjoy!

Nutritional values Press size: 1 bowl Calories: 388

Fat: 29 g

Carbohydrates: 14 g

Fiber: 8 g

Protein: 30 g

Prep: 5 minutes
Cooking time: 15 minutes Yield: 3 servings

Ingredients
1 pound ground beef
1 (9-ounce) package of raw coleslaw 2 spring onions, thinly sliced
1 tablespoon freshly grated peeled ginger 2 tablespoons of soy sauce
1 tablespoon of sriracha Optional black sesame seeds

Instructions
Prepare the sauce: Stir the soy sauce and sriracha together with a spoon in a small mixing bowl into a smooth mass. Put aside. Cook beef and cabbage: Cook ground beef in a large saucepan over medium heat until brown and crumbled, then spread the meat with a sturdy utensil, about 5 minutes. Leave beef and fat in the pan and stir in the coleslaw mix until the cabbage is limp and soft about 5 minutes.

Add finishing touch: reduce heat to medium-low. Stir in prepared sauce (soy sauce and sriracha) and ginger until well blended, about 1 minute. Turn off the heat. Stir in the chopped spring onions and garnish with sesame seeds if desired. Serve immediately while hot.

Nutritional values
Press size: 1 bowl
Calories: 388
Fat: 29 g
Carbohydrates: 14 g
Fiber: 8 g
Protein: 30 g

Preparation time: 10 minutes Cooking time: 10 minutes Total time: 20 minutes Servings: 4 people

Ingredients
1 pound of cauliflower 4 ounces of sour cream
1 cup of grated cheddar cheese
2 slices of bacon cooked and crumbled 2 tablespoons chopped chives
3 tablespoons of butter
1/4 teaspoon of garlic powder Salt and pepper to taste

Instructions
Cut the cauliflower into florets and place in a microwave-safe bowl. Add 2 tablespoons of water and cover with cling film. Microwave for 5-8 minutes, depending on your microwave, until tender and cooked through. Drain the excess water and leave it uncovered for a minute or two. (You can also steam your cauliflower the conventional way. You may need to squeeze a little water out of the cauliflower after cooking.)

Add the cauliflower to a food processor and process until fluffy. Add the butter, garlic powder, and sour cream and process until it resembles the consistency of mashed potatoes. Remove the mashed cauliflower from a bowl and add most of the chives, saving some to add on top later. Add half of the cheddar cheese and mix by hand. Season with salt and pepper.

Cover the loaded cauliflower with the remaining cheese, remaining chives, and bacon. Return to the microwave to melt the cheese or place the cauliflower under the broiler for a few minutes.

For 4 persons with 4.6 g net carbohydrates.
Nutritional values Calories: 298kcal Carbohydrates: 7.4 g
Protein: 11.6 g Fat: 24.6 g Saturated fat: 15.4 g

5 minutes preparation
15 minutes of cooking time Portions 4

Ingredients
11/3 lbs pork belly
2 tbsp tamari soy sauce 1 tbsp rice vinegar
2 cloves of garlic
3 oz. butter or coconut oil 1 pound Brussels sprouts
½ leeks
Salt and ground black pepper

Instructions
Cut the pork belly into bite-sized pieces. Rinse and trim the Brussels sprouts. Cut into halves or quarters, depending on their size. Put the pork in a saucepan and put it on medium heat. Fry until golden brown. Crush the garlic cloves and add them along with the Brussels sprouts and butter. Fry until the sprouts start to turn golden brown.

Mix soy sauce and rice vinegar in a small bowl and put it in the pan. Season with salt and pepper. Finally, sprinkle with thinly sliced leeks. Stir everything together and serve.

Nutritional values
Net carbs: 3% (7 g)
Fiber: 5 g
Fats: 89% (97 g)
Protein: 8% (19 g)
kcal : 993

91. Easy salmon patties without eggs

Preparation time: 10 minutes Cooking time: 10 minutes Total time: 20 minutes Servings: 6 patties

Ingredients
6 tablespoons of water
2 tablespoons of golden flaxseed flour
18 oz wild pink salmon (about 3 cans), drained well (see notes)
½ cup of almond flour
1/2 cup fresh parsley, chopped 1 shallot, finely chopped
1 green onion, sliced 1 teaspoon of salt
1 teaspoon of garlic powder
½ teaspoon of dill
¼ teaspoon of black pepper 2 tablespoons of lime juice 2 tablespoons of olive oil

Instructions
Add flaxseed meal and water to a small bowl and stir. Let rest for 5 minutes to thicken. Peel the salmon in a medium bowl. Add almond flour, parsley, shallot, green onion, salt, garlic powder, dill, black pepper, lime juice, and the flaxseed mixture. Mix until well incorporated.

Shape into 6 patties. I use a 1/2 cup measuring cup to portion the mixture and to make sure all the patties are the same size.
Heat olive oil over medium heat in a nonstick frying pan. Fry the patties for 4 to 5 minutes on each side until golden and crispy.

Serve with cilantro lime cauliflower rice, if desired

Nutritional values
Calories: 232kcal | Carbohydrates: 4 g | Protein: 22g | Fat: 14 g | Saturated fat: 1 g | Cholesterol: 70 mg | Sodium: 717 mg

92. Curried Riced Cauliflower with Shrimp

Preparation time 5 min Cooking time 15 min Total time 20 min
Servings: 4

Ingredients
1 bag of Green Giant Riced Cauliflower frozen 1 onion chopped
1/2 red pepper chopped 2 cloves Garlic chopped
1 pound uncooked shrimp peeled and gutted 2 tablespoons of chopped parsley
3/4 cup low- sodium chicken stock 2 teaspoons Curry powder
1 teaspoon of cumin
1 teaspoon of smoked paprika Half a lime juice
2 teaspoons Extra virgin olive oil Salt + pepper to taste

Instructions
Heat the olive oil in a frying pan over medium heat. Add the onions and pepper. Season with salt and pepper and cook for 3-4 minutes or until softened. Add the garlic and cook 1 minute more Pour the entire bag of Green Giant Riced Cauliflower into the pan. Mix with a wooden spoon

Add the cumin, curry, and smoked paprika. Stir. When everything is combined, add the chicken stock. Reduce heat to medium-low. Season the shrimps with salt and pepper. Place them in the cauliflower rice. Cover and cook for 2-3 minutes. Do not overcook the shrimp. Cover, add the parsley, and squeeze the lime juice over it. Stir and check for spices. Remove from the heat and enjoy!

Nutritional values
Calories 183 Calories from Fat 36
% Daily Value Fats 4g6%
Cholesterol 285 mg 95%
Sodium 919 mg 40%
Potassium 247 mg 7%
Carbohydrates 8 g 3% Fiber 3g13%

Preparation time: 10 minutes Cooking time: 20 minutes Total time: 30 minutes Servings 4

Ingredients
4 salmon fillets Gremolata
2 cloves of garlic
1/4 cup parsley leaves 1 lemon, grated
1 cup of almond flour 1 tbsp olive oil
Salt Pepper
Roasted Vegetables (optional) 1 bunch of asparagus
1 cup of cherry tomatoes 1 tbsp olive oil
Salt Pepper

Instructions
Heat your oven to 350F for a convection oven, 380F for non-convection oven. Mix the garlic, parsley and almond flour in a blender or food processor, then stir in the lemon zest. Place the salmon fillets on a greased or parchment-lined baking tray. Season the salmon fillets with salt and pepper, brush or spray with a little oil and gently press the Gremolata crumb mixture on top. If you are using the optional vegetables for roasting alongside the salmon, simply toss them in a little oil, place them around the salmon on the baking tray and season with salt and pepper. Bake for 15-   20 minutes until the fish is cooked through and the top is golden brown.

Nutritional Values
Calories 494 Calories from Fat 279
% Daily Value
Fats 31g48%
Saturated fat 3g 19%
Cholesterol 93 mg 31%

Preparation time: 20 minutes Cooking time: 10 minutes Total time: 30 minutes Servings 4

Ingredients

2 summer squash

2 tbsp unsalted butter 1/4 cup of chicken stock

2 tbsp lemon juice or white wine 1/8 tsp red chili flakes

Salt and pepper to taste

1 pound of shrimp stripped

2 tbsp parsley finely chopped 1 toe garlic minced

Instructions

Cut the summer squash into noodle shapes with a spiral cutter. Divide the noodles over kitchen paper. Sprinkle with salt and let rest for 15-30 minutes. Blot off the excess moisture or wring it lightly with dry paper towels. In a container or pan, melt butter over medium heat and sauté garlic. Add chicken stock, lemon juice (or wine), and red chili flakes. Bring to a boil and add the shrimp. Simmer until shrimp start to turn pink and reduce heat to low. Taste the sauce and mix in salt and pepper to taste. Add the summer squash noodles and parsley to the pan and mix the shrimp distribute to cover the noodles and sauce. Remove from heat and serve.

Nutritional values

Serving Size: 489g (~1/2 of the recipe)

Calories: 334kcal

Carbohydrates: 8.49 g

Protein: 48.4 g

Fat: 13.1 g Saturated fat: 7.49 g

Servings: 1

Ingredients

2 cups of mixed greens 1 large tomato, diced

¼ cup of fresh parsley, chopped

¼ cup of fresh mint, chopped 10 large kalamata olives, pitted 1 small zucchini, cut lengthwise

½ avocado cut into cubes 1 green onion, sliced

1 can chop light tuna in water, drained 1 tablespoon of extra virgin olive oil

1 tbsp balsamic vinegar

¼ teaspoon of Himalayan salt or fine sea salt

¾ tsp freshly cracked black pepper

Instructions

Grill the zucchini slices on both sides in a sizzling cast-iron skillet grill pan (or on a very hot grill). Remove from pan and let cool for a few minutes. Cut into bite-sized pieces. Place all ingredients in a large mixing bowl and stir gently until well blended. Serve immediately.

Nutritional values

Serving Size: 489g (~1/2 of the recipe)

Calories: 334kcal

Carbohydrates: 8.49 g

Protein: 48.4 g

Fat: 13.1 g Saturated fat: 7.49 g

Preparation Time: 10 Minutes Cooking Time: 20 Minutes Total Time: 30 Minutes Servings: 4 Persons

Ingredients
4 salmon fillets without bones Salt and pepper to taste
1 pound asparagus ends trimmed
1 lemon, thinly sliced (plus extra wedges for garnish) 1/2 cup butter, at room temperature
3 teaspoons Italian herbs or Provencal herbs see note 3 teaspoons of minced garlic
Fresh thyme or parsley, for garnish

Instructions
Season the salmon generously with salt and pepper on both sides. Place a salmon fillet and 1/4 of the asparagus in the center of a 12 "x 12" piece of foil. Repeat with the remaining salmon and asparagus on 3 other pieces of foil. Slide lemon slices under the salmon and asparagus.

Mix in a small bowl of butter, Italian seasoning, and garlic. Spoon large dollops of herb butter over the salmon and asparagus. Wrap the foil tightly around the salmon and asparagus, making sure to seal the ends tightly so that the juices and butter don't run out during cooking. Grill over medium heat for 6-8 minutes on each side, OR bake at 400 degrees for 20 minutes, until the asparagus is tender and the salmon flaky. Drizzle fresh lemon juice over the top and serve immediately.

Nutritional values
Serving Size: 489g (~1/2 of the recipe)
Calories: 334kcal
Carbohydrates: 8.49 g
Protein: 48.4 g
Fat: 13.1 g Saturated fat: 7.49 g

97. Mediterranean Roasted Cabbage Steaks With Basil Pesto & Feta

Yield: 5 Servings Preparation
Time: 5 Minutes Cooking
Time: 20 Minutes

Ingredients

1 small head of cabbage, cut into "steaks" 4 oz Basil Pesto
1 cup of grated Parmesan cheese 2 oz feta cheese, crumbled
2 small tomatoes, sliced
5-6 marinated artichoke halves
1 tablespoon of Mediterranean herbs

Fresh basil, for garnish
OPTIONAL TOPPINGS include olives, mozzarella, mushrooms, roasted red peppers, etc.

Instructions

Heat the oven to 400 and spray a large baking sheet with nonstick cooking spray. Place the cabbage in a single layer on the baking sheet so that the edges touch. Spread pesto on the steak halves and be generous as much will melt in the cabbage folds. Cover with cheese and tomato and cook until the edges of the cabbage are crisp and all the cheese is bubbly. In 20 minutes. Sprinkle with herbs and basil. Serve HOT with an extra scoop of Pesto for dipping!

Nutritional Value

Calories 243
16 g Carbohydrates
16 g Protein
12 g fats

Preparation time 5

minutes Cooking time 20

minutes Total time 25

minutes Servings 4

Ingredients

Rice

12 ounces Cauliflower rice

1 teaspoon toasted sesame oil 1 teaspoon coconut Aminos

Vegetables

1 cup of Matchstick carrots

1 cup bean sprouts (omit for strict paleo) 1 cup cucumber (julienned)

2 cups of spinach

4 medium spring onions

1 teaspoon toasted sesame oil (divided) Sea salt (to taste)

Other toppings 2-4 large eggs Kimchi Sriracha

Click to convert between US and Metric measurements: Common in the US - metric

Instructions

More TIPS on this paleo recipe in the post above! Heat a skillet over medium heat with 1 teaspoon of sesame oil. Add the cauliflower rice and cook until soft and toasted, about 5 minutes. Drizzle with coconut Aminos. Remove and divide between two bowls. Wipe the pan and add 1/4 teaspoon of sesame oil and carrots. Bake for about 30 seconds until soft. Add a pinch of salt. Remove from pan and set aside. Repeat with bean sprouts. In the same pan, add half a teaspoon of sesame oil and spinach after removing the Brussels sprouts. Cook for about 1 minute or until wilted. Grill the spring onions over high heat until charred. I just put them over my gas burner, but you can also use a regular grill or grill pan. See the comments for another option. In a small ceramic or well-seasoned cast-iron skillet, fry the eggs with a little sesame oil until the egg white is crisp and firm, but the yolk is still runny. Divide the vegetables between the two plates, cover with eggs, kimchi, cucumbers, and the grilled or sliced spring onions. Serve with Sriracha.

Nutritional Value

Amount per serving. Serving size in recipe notes above Calories 207
Fat 9g
Protein 12g
Total carbohydrates 22g Net carbohydrates 15g Fiber 7g
Sugar 10g

99.   Vegan Thai curry

Preparation time 5 minutes Cooking time 15 minutes
Total time 20 minutes Servings 4

Ingredients

1 packet of tofu 454 g, cut into 16 cubes. 2 peppers (red and green)
cut into strips 2 tbsp coconut oil
1 tbsp tomato paste
1 tin 15 oz coconut milk full fat 2 tsp chili flakes
1 teaspoon of Thai curry paste 1 tbsp almond butter
Piece of ginger peeled the size of a thumb Cut 1 stalk of lemongrass
into 3 pieces
1 clove of garlic
1/4 cup of soy sauce

Instructions

Heat a pan over medium heat and melt your coconut oil. Chop your
ginger and garlic and put them in the pan. Add your bell pepper
strips and lemongrass pieces. Stir for 30 seconds and add your
coconut milk and cooling flakes. Stir again. Add your soy sauce, Thai
curry paste, tomato paste, and almond butter. Stir for 1 minute and
add your Tofu cubes. Let your curry cook for 5-10 minutes, or until
the sauce thickens and remove from heat. Serve with chopped
cilantro and green onions to add some freshness to the dish.

Nutritional Value

Calories: 318 Kcal
Carbohydrates: 9.1 g
Protein: 12 g
Fat: 27.1 g
Fiber: 2.1 g

Preparation time: 20
minutes Cooking time: 10
minutes Total time: 30
minutes Yield: 6 tacos

Ingredients

Portobello mushrooms
1 pound (450 g) of portobello mushrooms
1/4 cup (60 g) spicy harissa, or use a mild harissa 3 tablespoons of olive oil, divided
1 teaspoon of cumin powder 1 teaspoon of onion powder

6 collard green leaves
Guacamole
2 medium ripe avocados
2 tablespoons of diced tomatoes
2 tablespoons of chopped red onion
1 1/2 to 2 tablespoons of lemon or lime juice Pinch of salt
1 tablespoon of chopped cilantro
Optional toppings Cashew cream Chopped tomatoes Chopped cilantro

Instructions

Remove the stem from the portobello mushrooms. Rinse and pat the mushrooms dry. Mix harissa, 1 1/2 tablespoons of olive oil, cumin, and onion powder in a bowl. Brush each mushroom with the harissa mixture, making sure to cover the edges of the mushroom as well. Let the mushrooms marinate for 15 minutes. While the mushrooms are marinating, prepare guacamole. Halve and stone the avocados and scoop out the pulp. Puree avocados and mix chopped tomatoes, red onion, lemon (or lime) juice, salt, and cilantro. Put aside. Rinse kale. Cut off the tough stems and set aside. When the mushrooms are done marinating, heat 1 1/2 tablespoons of olive oil in a skillet or sauté the pan over medium heat. Place the portobello mushrooms in the pan and cook for 3 minutes. Flip and cook for 2 to 3 more minutes. Each side should be brown. Turn off the heat and let the mushrooms rest for 2 to 3 minutes before slicing them. Take a green leaf and fill it with a few slices of portobello. Add guacamole, chopped tomatoes, cashew cream, and cilantro to taste.

Nutritional Value

For 6 Tacos, Amount for 2 Tacos: Calories: 405,
Total Fat 34.4g, Saturated Fat: 5g, Sodium: 226mg, Cholesterol: 0mg

CPSIA information can be obtained
at www.ICGtesting.com
Printed in the USA
BVHW091043240221
600902BV00003B/653